KT-103-224

O A P L
OXFORD AMERICAN PSYCHIATRY LIBRARY

Adherence to Mental Health Treatment

O A P L
OXFORD AMERICAN PSYCHIATRY LIBRARY

Adherence to Mental Health Treatment

Peter F. Buckley, MD
Department of Psychiatry & Health Behavior
Medical College of Georgia, Augusta, GA

Adriana Foster, MD
Department of Psychiatry & Health Behavior
Medical College of Georgia, Augusta, GA

Nick C. Patel, PharmD, PhD
LifeSynch, Inc. Fort Worth, TX
Department of Psychiatry & Health Behavior
Medical College of Georgia, Augusta, GA

Anastasia Wermert, BA
Department of Psychiatry & Health Behavior
Medical College of Georgia, Augusta, GA

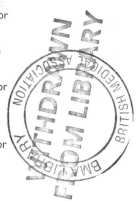

OXFORD
UNIVERSITY PRESS
2009

OXFORD
UNIVERSITY PRESS

Oxford University Press, Inc., publishes works that further
Oxford University's objective of excellence
in research, scholarship, and education.

Oxford New York
Auckland Cape Town Dar es Salaam Hong Kong Karachi
Kuala Lumpur Madrid Melbourne Mexico City Nairobi
New Delhi Shanghai Taipei Toronto

With offices in
Argentina Austria Brazil Chile Czech Republic France Greece
Guatemala Hungary Italy Japan Poland Portugal Singapore
South Korea Switzerland Thailand Turkey Ukraine Vietnam

Copyright © 2009 by Oxford University Press, Inc.

Published by Oxford University Press, Inc.
198 Madison Avenue, New York, New York 10016
www.oup.com

Oxford is a registered trademark of Oxford University Press

Library of Congress Cataloging-in-Publication Data

Adherence to mental health treatment/Peter F. Buckley ... [et al.].
    p. ; cm.—(Oxford American psychiatry library)
Includes bibliographical references and index.
ISBN 978-0-19-538433-8 (standard edition)—1. Psychotherapy patients.
2. Patient compliance. 3. Psychotropic drugs. I. Buckley, Peter, 1943- II. Series.
[DNLM: 1. Mentally Ill Persons—psychology. 2. Treatment Refusal—psychology.
3. Mental Disorders—drug therapy. 4. Mental Disorders—psychology.
WM 29.5 P9736 2009]
RC483.P756 2009
616.89'14—dc22   2008043009

9 8 7 6 5 4 3 2 1
Printed in the United States of America
on acid-free paper

Preface

Failing to complete a simple course of antibiotics or forgetting to take medications as prescribed by the doctor is a remarkably common human experience. This experience and its impact upon disease management are magnified in chronic illnesses. For people with chronic medical illnesses, nonadherence with treatment substantially adds to the burden as well as poorer long-term outcome in these conditions. For people with mental illness, the frequency and impact of poor adherence to treatment are even more pronounced than in other medical conditions. Adherence to treatment is further undermined by the impairments in insight that often accompany mental illness. Much has been written about this topic, often in disease-specific publications and in the overall context of management of a particular condition. However, the topic of adherence itself is so common and complex across mental illnesses that it merits review in its own right. In this book we summarize the current knowledge about adherence to treatment in mental illness. We review in detail how adherence is a common obstacle to care. We also point to the commonality of findings throughout the literature about treatment adherence in mental illness. In doing so, we include findings in other disease conditions of relevance to clinicians who deal with a variety of disease circumstances on a daily basis. We also have included direct comments of consumers. The book includes concise, practical information for clinicians on a key topic that all of us struggle with. The data are presented in a "ready-to-use" manner using algorithms, diagrams, tables, and figures to convey the clinical information and guidance to the clinicians.

The authors of this book have used many sources and can make no guarantees that all information provided is accurate, current, and without error. Readers should consult primary sources provided in the appendix and toolbox for the most up-to-date published product and lab information. The authors and the publishers do not accept responsibility or legal liability for any errors in the text or for the misuse or misapplication of material in this work.

Contents

Chapter 1

Adherence and the societal burden of mental illness

Failing to complete a simple course of antibiotics or forgetting to take medications as prescribed by the doctor is a remarkably common human experience. This experience and its impact on disease management are magnified in chronic illnesses. For people with chronic medical illnesses, nonadherence with treatment substantially adds to the burden and leads to poorer long-term outcomes in these conditions. For people with mental illness, the frequency and impact of poor adherence to treatment are even more pronounced than in other medical conditions. Adherence to treatment is further undermined by the impairments in insight that often accompany mental illness.

Most recently, the seminal Clinical Antipsychotic Trials of Intervention Effectiveness (CATIE) study showed that 74% patients with psychotic illness discontinued antipsychotic treatment before 18 months,[1] underlining the point that sticking to the treatment regimen is challenging for people with long-term mental illness. A similarly high discontinuation rate was reported in a comparable first-episode study of antipsychotic treatment tolerability and efficacy.[2] This suggests that medication nonadherence is a major consideration, even at the beginning of treatment. Moreover, medication nonadherence rates for psychiatric conditions are generally worse than for other medical conditions, as will be discussed further in Chapter 2.

The scope of the problem

What makes this such an issue is the disproportionate impact of mental illness on society. If you consider mortality as an indicator of severe impact, then cardiovascular illness, which accounts for over one third of deaths, is the most devastating. However, if you take a broader perspective and include lifelong disability and also premature mortality, then psychiatric conditions constitute a major burden to society.[3]

Depression

In the Global Burden of Diseases, an economic study commissioned by the World Health Organization, Murray and Lopez found that mental illnesses were responsible for almost 25% of all the disability in developed countries.[3] Unipolar depression was the most disabling condition, which is likely because depression and other psychiatric conditions are remarkably common (Fig. 1.1).

Depression exerts an inordinate personal and familial burden. It is associated with unemployment and poorer medical outcomes. In a meta-analysis of the effects

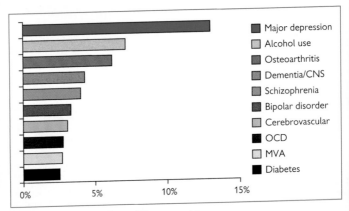

Figure 1.1 The impact of mental illness on society.

of anxiety and depression on patient adherence, DiMatteo and colleagues found a significant relationship between depression and nonadherence with treatment recommendations in patients with a variety of medical conditions.[4] Overall, they found that depressed patients were three times more likely to be noncompliant with treatment regimens than nondepressed patients. Depression is even more common in chronic medical conditions (e.g., diabetes, cardiovascular illnesses), and it is associated with treatment nonadherence and poorer outcomes for these conditions as well. Depression has been consistently identified as a risk factor for morbidity and mortality in patients with coronary heart disease. Recent research has identified treatment nonadherence as a likely contributor to such adverse cardiovascular outcomes in depressed patients. A 2005 cross-sectional study of 940 outpatients with stable coronary heart disease found a significant association between depression and medication nonadherence. Depressed participants were more likely than nondepressed participants to report not taking medication as prescribed, forgetting to take medication, and purposely skipping medication.[5] A recent study by Gonzalez and colleagues suggests that even subclinical depressive symptoms are associated with poorer self-care and medication adherence in type 2 diabetics.[6] Depression has also been implicated as a strong predictor of nonadherence with antipsychotics in patients experiencing their first episode of psychosis.[7]

Depression is also, of course, strongly associated with suicide. Suicide accounts for more violent deaths worldwide than either homicide or war-related deaths. It is the 11th most common cause of death in America, and the fourth leading cause of death in young adolescents.

Medication nonadherence and health beliefs

Sick role, personal model of illness

We have been unsure how to attribute this phenomenon of "not taking medication." It is a major consideration because we will undermine our therapeutic alliance and risk being pejorative to patients if we characterize this as "their fault." It is, of course, much more complex than that. Fundamentally, aspects of the "sick role," medical sociology, and expectations of the person who is sick are all of great relevance here. Parsons illuminated the concept of the "sick role" in which individuals adopt behaviors and expectations that receive societal sanction and support (Table 1.1).[8]

More recently, Leventhal and colleagues elaborated the components of a personal model of illness (Table 1.2).

Leventhal's model emphasizes the core beliefs that patients have and their impact on illness management.[9,10] These beliefs are informed by a variety of sources and are shaped by their experiences. This model espouses an approach involving "weighing up all the odds" where the patient gets to decide how priorities stack up. People have an individualized view of illness and their capacity to cope based on their beliefs about the illness and the extent to which they can control their own destiny. This health beliefs model has been applied in medicine, especially in preventive medicine, where the person's choices and behaviors can determine his or her health outcomes.[11] Brown and colleagues have also examined the role of health beliefs in depression. In a study of outpatients with depression, acceptance and religious beliefs were found to explain in part the level of functioning.[12] Such approaches have wide applicability to other mental conditions and to our understanding of medication adherence.

Culture and ethnicity

Culture is also a powerful determinant of a patient's perception about illness. In the classic study by Zborowski at a Veterans Affairs (VA) hospital examining the experience of pain among patients of different cultures, patients of Jewish culture had a more stoic acceptance of pain, while Italian patients were more concerned with obtaining relief for their pain.[13] There are similar recent examples in the psychopharmacology of mood disorders. In the Systematic Treatment Enhancement Program for Bipolar Disorder (STEP-BD), Gonzales and colleagues reported that Latin patients had fewer treatment visits, lower medication adherence rates, and more frequent use of religious supports than European Americans.[14] Fleck and colleagues examined medication nonadherence among African American and Caucasian patients with bipolar disorder.[15] African American patients viewed nonadherence more in the context of patient-related experiences, relating fears

Table 1.1 Key Components of Parson's "Sick Role"[8]

- Individual is exempt from usual social responsibilities
- Individual lacks voluntary control over illness
- Individual is expected to perceive condition as undesirable, desire to get well
- Individual is expected to seek competent help

Table 1.2 Common Components of Leventhal's Personal Model of Illness

Identification	How patient defines the illness/symptoms
Cause	Beliefs about what caused the illness/symptoms
Timeline	Expected duration of illness/symptoms
Consequences	Expected outcome of illness/symptoms
Perceived controllability	Beliefs about various treatment efficacies

Adapted with permission from Delgado (2000)[9].

that the medications may be addictive and that the medications were themselves a powerful and stigmatizing symbol of mental illness.[15] Table 1.3 summarizes studies on ethnic and cultural assumptions about psychotropic medications.[14–21]

Role of families

Families also play a crucial role in shaping health beliefs. We see this in clinical practice when a family's perceptions and beliefs about a proposed trial of a new medication for their loved one has a powerful influence on whether the patient decides to accept the treatment. If a family member views the mental symptoms in more behaviorally based terms, then other nonmedical approaches will be emphasized and the role of medications may be perceived as ancillary. Conversely, families may attach great significance to medication treatments, thereby heightening the expectation that the medication might be a cure-all. Family support and

Table 1.3 Cultural Differences and Psychotropic Medications		
Ethnicity	**Psychosocial/Assumptions**	**Biological**
African Americans	More likely to have negative beliefs about antidepressants than whites (more agree "antidepressants are addictive" and less agree "antidepressants are effective")[16]	Higher percentage of CYP2D6*17, so may metabolize psychotropic medications more slowly[20,21]
	Less insight about illness[14]	
	Fewer mental health treatment visits[14]	
	Fear of addiction to medication[15]	
	Medication viewed as stigmatizing[15]	
	More likely to prefer counseling over medication for depression[17]	
Latinos	Fewer mental health treatment visits[14]	
	Lower adherence rates[14]	
	More frequent use of religious supports[14]	
	More likely to have negative beliefs about antidepressants than whites[16]	
Caucasian	View psychotropic medication use more favorably than minority patients[19]	
	More likely to consider medication to control panic episodes[18]	
	More likely to find antidepressant medication acceptable than African Americans[16]	
Asians		Higher percentage of CYP2C19 poor metabolizers, so may metabolize tricyclics and diazepam more slowly[21]

advocacy organizations such as the National Alliance for Mental Illness (NAMI) recognize this fundamental impact of relatives' beliefs and knowledge, and they invest heavily in appropriate educational support for family members.[22] Family support and education is a key component of care.[23] This aspect is also covered in Chapter 6.

Role of media and Internet

A person's health beliefs are also powerfully influenced by the broad environment in which he or she lives. America is a consumer-driven society. A disproportionate amount of the gross national product is spent on health care. Consumers expect that the latest treatments and technologies will be available. Direct-to-consumer (DTC) advertising on television and in magazines influences opinion on a wide scale and also directly affects the patient–clinician interactions.

Healy has written eloquently of the cultural shift regarding depression and its treatment after the powerful marketing of fluoxetine (Prozac) in the 1990s.[24] A decade later, antidepressant medications have been the subject of intense media attention because of a purported heightened risk of suicide during treatment. The highly publicized suicide "black box" warning on all antidepressant medications and associated treatment recommendations from the U.S. Food and Drug Administration (FDA) was followed by a sharp decline in prescriptions of these drugs for children.[25]

There is also a great public concern about giving any medications to children, given the effects they could have on development. For example, there is concern that giving stimulant drugs to children with attention-deficit/hyperactivity disorder (ADHD) could result in higher rates of substance abuse in adolescents.[26] Similar public concern emerged after widely publicized U.S. media coverage of an unproven association between the measles-mumps-rubella (MMR) vaccine and autism. During this time, there was an outbreak of measles in Indiana in 2005. Thirty-two of the 34 people affected were unvaccinated, and the primary reason given for this was concern for adverse events, specifically those related to media reports of the potential link between MMR and autism.[27]

It is not uncommon for the public to be "warned" about medical issues well in advance of scientific evidence to support such warnings. For example, the risk of diabetes mellitus during antipsychotic therapy was widely publicized in the lay press in advance of a clear and scientific appraisal of the strength of this association.[28]

The lay public has been well apprised of serious side effects of medications, and of course all of this forms the context in which any given patient considers the risk–benefit profile of prescribed medication, as well as whether he or she will take it or not. Ensuring the safety of the public from potentially harmful effects of medications is a daily theme in the media. The well-publicized story of rofecoxib (Vioxx) is an example, as it fueled public concern that other drugs in use might also be later considered dangerous.[29] Patients with mental illness are naturally very concerned about the potential side effects of medication. Sometimes they, too, harbor the concern (just like in the Vioxx story) that there is some unknown serious side effect associated with the drug that they are being asked to take. Moreover, the finding of the Institute of Medicine report that 44,000 to 98,000 deaths annually are attributable to medication-related errors has received widespread attention.[30] This provides "proof" that drugs can be harmful, and of course this further fuels the real concerns of patients about their medications.

The Internet has also emerged as a great source of information and opinion about mental illness and its treatments. Indeed, more Americans consult the Internet for information about mental illness than they do for any other condition.

Disease-specific Web sites, regulatory and pharmaceutical Web sites, blogs, and various other sources together form a diverse repertoire of knowledge, experience, and professional and lay opinions about any given treatment. These sources are of much more relevance today. Patients have ready access to information about medications. Some sources are more scientific, some are more lay, and some are skeptical of any medications. The person trying to inform himself or herself about medications has a wide range of choices, and the information offered will differ substantially from Web site to Web site.

In any case, the Internet and consumerism are now powerful determinants of today's health beliefs and information about medications.

Definitions of Adherence, compliance, and concordance

Terms used to describe medication nonadherence evoke emotional responses (Table 1.4). Until recently "noncompliance" was the term most commonly used to describe this phenomenon. In an era of consumerism, however, this term has fallen into disrepute and is considered pejorative as it devalues self-care and autonomy. "Adherence" holds similar, overly medicalized connotations. "Concordance" is slowly gaining favor as a term that is responsive to consumer needs and connotes joint decision making with the clinician. Rather than focusing on control and responsibility, it emphasizes the alignment between the patient's and the clinician's objectives.[31,32]

Consumerism

The notion of self-determinism also resonates with the recovery movement in psychiatry. Patients with mental illness are increasingly assuming greater responsibility for their care, and through this individuation process they are refocusing the goals of treatment toward what they consider to be more meaningful outcomes. In this scheme, the medical model is not necessarily put aside, but is

Table 1.4 Definitions of Adherence

Term	Definition[31]	Pros and Cons[32]
Compliance	The consistency and accuracy with which someone follows the regimen prescribed by a physician or other health professional	• Exaggerates control of physician • Suggests conformity to instructions is necessary to reach goals of therapy • Implies unilateral decision enforcement by physician • Noncompliance/nonadherence does not accurately distinguish differences in patients' medication-taking behaviors (i.e., patient who forgets to take an occasional pill versus a patient who rarely fills a prescription)
Adherence	The extent to which a patient continues an agreed-on mode of treatment without close supervision	
Concordance	A negotiated, shared agreement between clinician and patient concerning treatment regimen(s), outcomes, and behaviors	• Implies an alliance in decision making between patient and physician

it "relegated" and put in context of the person's overall life journey and struggle with illness.[33] The role of medications is still relevant, but more as a facilitator rather than as the bedrock of treatment. Also, terms like "compliance" or "adherence" are not well tolerated. Patients view medication as a means to an end—that is, the medication helps them remain stable and counteracts symptoms, while their "real" recovery from mental illness is defined by other attributes such as personal strength, hope, spirituality, family support, or social support.

For others, relying on medication is seen as running counter to the recovery model. The patient feels that he or she can "go it alone" and that medications are more of a "crutch." This viewpoint is naturally more likely to be associated with poor adherence to prescribed medications.

There is an increasing desire among patients to be more involved in decisions concerning their care. Shared decision making is "a collaborative process between a client and a practitioner, both of whom recognize one another as experts and work together to exchange information and clarify values in order to arrive at health care decisions."[34] A recent pilot study of a shared decision-making intervention in a psychiatric outpatient medicine clinic showed evidence that consultations were more focused on a patient's specific wants and needs and that clients felt more empowered to take part in treatment-related decisions.[34]

References

1. Lieberman JA, Stroup TS, McEvoy JP, et al. Effectiveness of antipsychotic drugs in patients with chronic schizophrenia. N Engl J Med. 2005;353:1209–1223.

2. McEvoy JP, Lieberman JA, Perkins DO, et al. Efficacy and tolerability of olanzapine, quetiapine, and risperidone in the treatment of early psychosis: a randomized, double-blind 52-week comparison. Am J Psychiatry. 2007; 164:1050–1060.

3. Murray CJ, Lopez AD. Evidence-based health policy-lessons from the Global Burden of Disease Study. Science. 1996;274:740–743.

4. DiMatteo MR, Lepper HS, Croghan TW. Depression is a risk factor for non-compliance with medical treatment: meta-analysis of the effects of anxiety and depression on patient adherence. Arch Intern Med. 2007;160:2101–2107.

5. Gehi A, Haas D, Pipkin S, Whooley MA. Depression and medication adherence in outpatients with coronary heart disease: findings from the Heart and Soul Study. Arch Intern Med. 2005;165:2508–2513.

6. Gonzalez JS, Safren SA, Cagliero E, et al. Depression, self-care and medication adherence in type 2 diabetes: relationships across the full range of symptom severity. Diabetes Care. 2007;30:2222–2227.

7. Perkins DO, Gu H, Weiden PJ, McEvoy JP, Hamer RM, Lieberman JA. Predictors of treatment discontinuation and medication nonadherence in patients recovering from a first episode of schizophrenia, schizophreniform disorder, or schizo-affective disorder: a randomized, double-blind, flexible-dose, multicenter study. J Clin Psychiatry. 2008;69:106–113.

8. Kaplan BS, Sadock VA. Comprehensive Textbook of Psychiatry, 7th ed. New York: Lippincott Williams & Wilkins; 2000:1533.

9. Delgado PL. Approaches to the enhancement of patient adherence to antidepressant medication treatment. J Clin Psychiatry. 2000;61(Suppl 2):6–9.

10. Leventhal H, Nerenz DR. The assessment of illness cognition. In: Karoly P, ed. Management Strategies in Health Psychology. New York: John Wiley and Sons; 1985:517–554.

11. Orbell S, Hagger M, Brown V, Tidy J. Comparing two theories of health behavior: a prospective study of noncompletion of treatment following cervical cancer screening. *Health Psychol.* 2006;25:604–615.

12. Brown C, Battista DR, Sereika SM, Bruehlman RD, Dunbar-Jacob J, Thase ME. Primary care patients' personal illness models for depression: relationship to coping behavior and functional disability. *Gen Hosp Psychiatry.* 2007;29:492–500.

13. Encandela JA. Social science and the study of pain since Zborowski: a need for a new agenda. *Soc Sci Med.* 1993;36:783–791.

14. Gonzalez JM, Thompson P, Escamilla M, et al. Treatment characteristics and illness burden among European Americans, African Americans and Latinos in the first 2,000 patients of the systematic treatment enhancement program for bipolar disorder. *Psychopharmacol Bull.* 2007;40:31–46.

15. Fleck DE, Keck PE, Corey KB, Strakowski SM. Factors associated with medication adherence in African American and white patients with bipolar disorder. *J Clin Psychiatry.* 2005;66:646–652.

16. Cooper LA, Gonzales JJ, Gallo JJ, et al. The acceptability of treatment for depression among African-American, Hispanic, and white primary care patients. *Med Care.* 2003;41:479–489.

17. Dwight-Johnson M, Sherbourne C, Liao D, Wells KB. Treatment preferences among depressed primary care patients. *J Gen Intern Med.* 2000;15:527–534.

18. Hazlett-Stevens H, Craske MG, Roy-Byrne PP, Sherbourne CD, Stein MB, Bystritsky A. Predictors of willingness to consider medication and psychosocial treatment for panic disorder in primary care patients. *Gen Hosp Psychiatry.* 2002;24:316–321.

19. Wagner AW, Bystritsky A, Russo JE, et al. Beliefs about psychotropic medication and psychotherapy among primary care patients with anxiety disorders. *Depress Anxiety.* 2005;21:99–105.

20. Bradford LD, Gaedigk A, Leeder JS. High frequency of CYP2D6 poor and "intermediate" metabolizers in black populations: a review and preliminary data. *Psychopharmacol Bull.* 1998;34:797–804.

21. De Leon J, Armstrong SC, Cozza KL. Clinical guidelines for psychiatrists for the use of pharmacogenetic testing for CYP450 2D6 and CYP450 2C19. *Psychosomatics.* 2006;47:75–85.

22. National Alliance on Mental Illness. http://www.nami.org. Accessed Aug. 10, 2008.

23. Cohen AN, Glynn SM, Murray-Swank AB, et al. The family forum: directions for the implementation of family psychoeducation for severe mental illness. *Psychiatr Serv.* 2008;59:40–48.

24. Healy D. Psychopharmacology and the ethics of resource allocation. *Br J Psychiatry.* 1993;162:23–29.

25. Nemeroff CB, Kalali A, Keller MB, et al. Impact of publicity concerning pediatric suicidality data on physician practice patterns in the United States. *Arch Gen Psychiatry.* 2007;64:466–472.

26. Volkow ND, Swanson JM. Does childhood treatment of ADHD with stimulant medication affect substance abuse in adulthood? *Am J Psychiatry.* 2008; 165:553–555.

27. Parker AA, Staggs W, Dayan GH, et al. Implications of a 2005 measles outbreak in Indiana for sustained elimination of measles in the United States. *N Engl J Med.* 2006;355:447–455.

28. Goode E. 3 Schizophrenia Drugs May Raise Diabetes Risk, Study Says. *New York Times.* http://query.nytimes.com/gst/fullpage.html?res=9D06E5DF1239F936A15 75BC0A9659C8B63&scp=1&sq=schizophrenia+drugs+may+raise+diabetes+ri sk&st=nyt. Accessed July 1, 2008.

29. Waxman HA. The lessons of Vioxx—drug safety and sales. *N Engl J Med.* 2005;352:2576.

30. Kohn LT, Corrigan JM, Donaldson MS, Committee on Quality of Health Care in America, Institute of Medicine. *To Err Is Human: Building A Safer Health System.* Washington, DC: National Academy Press; 2000:1.

31. *Stedman's Medical Dictionary,* 28th ed. Baltimore: Lippincott Williams & Wilkins; 2006.

32. Steiner JF, Earnest MA. The language of medication-taking. *Ann Intern Med.* 2000;132:926–930.

33. Frese FJ, Stanley J, Kress K, Vogel-Scibilia S. Integrating evidence-based practices and the recovery model. *Psychiatr Serv.* 2001;52:1462–1468.

34. Deegan, PE, Rapp C, Holter M, Riefer M. Best practices: a program to support shared decision making in an outpatient psychiatric medication clinic. *Psychiatr Serv.* 2008;59:603–605.

Chapter 2

Rates of nonadherence in psychiatric disorders

How big is the problem?

Does medicine, when taken, control psychiatric illness?

There is clear evidence that adherence to pharmacological therapy helps treat medical and psychiatric illness effectively. Each 10% increase in oral diabetes medication adherence is associated with a 0.1% decrease in glycosylated hemoglobin (HbA1C). Human immunodeficiency virus (HIV) viral load correlates closely with highly active antiretroviral therapy (HAART) adherence level: for adherence levels of more than 95%, over 80% of patients have an undetectable viral load, whereas if adherence falls below 70%, only 30% patients have an undetectable viral load. Aspirin reduces the risk of stroke by 22%, and warfarin reduces the risk of stroke by 62%.

Psychiatric illness responds to medication as well. A group of patients with recurrent depression who took part in a 3-year trial of treatment with imipramine and interpersonal therapy then participated in a 2-year randomized trial of active medication versus placebo.[1] Patients randomized to imipramine continued to show a significant prophylactic effect for the additional 2-year period compared to those on placebo. Among patients with bipolar I disorder followed for 10 years, the suicide rate was 5.2-fold higher in patients who were poorly adherent compared to those highly adherent to lithium.[2] Rates of relapse in schizophrenia are consistently lower across studies of patients treated with antipsychotics continuously compared with intermittent therapy (a strategy of antipsychotic discontinuation in stable outpatients attempting to mitigate the risk of adverse effects) over the same period (Fig. 2.1).[3]

According to Robinson and colleagues,[4] antipsychotic medication significantly reduces the risk of relapse within 5 years of recovery from the first episode of schizophrenia. In contrast, gender, duration of psychosis before treatment, baseline symptoms, presence of residual symptoms after initial episode, or presence of adverse effects during treatment are not related to the rate of relapse.

Treatment adherence in general medical illness

Infectious disease

A multinational patient survey of nonadherence with antibiotic therapy for acute community infections found that 22.3% of patients admitted nonadherence.

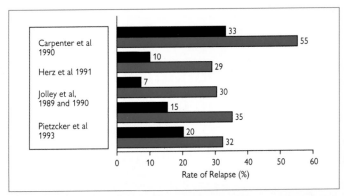

Figure 2.1 Rates of relapse in patients with schizophrenia after 1 year of continuous or intermittent maintenance therapy in five studies. Black bars represent continuous treatment and shaded bars intermittent treatment. Most patients had had more than one prior psychotic episode. The number of patients in each group in these studies ranged from 27 to 121. Adapted from Kane JM. Schizophrenia. *N Engl J Med.* 1996;334:34–41, with permission from the *New England Journal of Medicine.*

Thirteen percent of the homeless or marginally housed persons with HIV were found to be nonadherent to antiretroviral therapy, with adherence defined as taking less than 80% of the highly active antiretroviral treatment medication. Provider and patient assessment of adherence are both significantly higher than adherence measured by unannounced pill count.[5]

Hypertension and cardiovascular disease

Forty to 50% of patients with cardiovascular disease fail to follow prescribed regimens. In chronic conditions (e.g., coronary artery disease, hypertension, and post-acute coronary syndromes), adherence declines markedly after just 6 months of therapy.[6] In a large U.S. VA study,[7] antihypertensive adherence, measured with prescription fill records, varied between 78% for thiazide diuretics and 84% for angiotensin receptor blockers, while depression (as well as race) was a predictor for nonadherence. As stress theory has penetrated psychosomatic medicine, we have learned that the natural course of gastrointestinal, cardiovascular, respiratory, and endocrine disorders (among others) is highly influenced by psychosocial factors. For example, self-reported nonadherence was more common (14%) in depressed patients compared with those without depression (5%) in a cohort of over 900 patients with stable coronary heart disease.

Diabetes

Health behaviors important to persons with diabetes include self-monitoring of blood glucose, which can slow progression of diabetes complications. In 2000, according to the Behavioral Risk Surveillance System data from 47 U.S. states, the adherence with this measure varied between racial groups: 28% for Hispanics, 63% for African Americans, and 59% for non-Hispanic whites. Twenty percent of patients with type 2 diabetes meet criteria for probable major depression and 66.5% report at least some depressive symptoms. Major depression is significantly associated with poorer adherence to self-care measures like diet, exercise, and self-monitoring of blood sugar in diabetes. Cramer thoroughly evaluated adherence to medications for diabetes.[8]

Respiratory disease

Adherence with twice-daily dosing of inhaled steroids monitored electronically was found to be 63%.[9] Factors associated with poor adherence were number of formal education years, low household income, poor patient–clinician communication, and Spanish as primary language. In inner-city children with asthma, adherence monitored electronically with metered-dose inhalers was 28% at baseline but doubled after 1 month of a home-based intervention. Asthmatics with comorbid psychiatric illness have poorer asthma control and quality of life than those without symptoms of mental illness.

Several common themes emerge from this brief review: adherence depends on the level of symptoms and discomfort produced by the disease, socioeconomic status, and coping skills (Table 2.1). It appears that an "optimal" level of discomfort from the illness needs to be reached to motivate adherence. Pertinent to our field, mental illness is associated with poorer treatment adherence and poorer outcomes of general medical illness. Thus, one can conclude that treating mental illness symptoms can optimize general disease outcome (Fig. 2.2)

As summarized by Osterberg and Blaschke,[10] the nonadherence literature presents serious challenges. Firstly, adherence is variably defined and it is measured dichotomously (adherence versus nonadherence) or on a continuum. The dichotomous option uses a cutoff point chosen either empirically based on the nature of disease or after calculation of sensitivity and specificity. Other studies of adherence measure it on a continuum by assessing rates of adherence between 0% to over 100%, allowing the possibility that patients take more medication than recommended. Second, the methods of measuring nonadherence vary widely and include patient self-assessment, clinician assessment (unstructured or formal), with adherence rating scales (see Chapter 4), as well as electronic monitoring techniques and prescription fill records, which are generally used only in research studies (see Table 4.4 and Fig. 4.2). Understandably, these factors can have a paramount effect on the design and interpretation of results in studies of adherence.

Treatment adherence in psychiatric illness

It is challenging even to bring people into psychiatric treatment. No-show rates for the initial mental health appointment were 32% in Denmark,[11] 25% in Spain,[12] and 20% in the U.S. military.[13] Nonadherence rates for the initial appointment vary from approximately 18% in public health care in England to 50% for psychiatric consultations in a primary care clinic in the United States. Mild level of distress,

Table 2.1 Nonadherence Rate for Chronic Illnesses

	Coronary Heart Disease[6]	Hypertension[7]	Diabetes Type[28]	Asthma[9]	HIV[5]
Medication nonadherence rate	40–50%[a]	16–22%[b]	Oral hypoglycemic agents: 7–64%[a] Insulin: 37%[a]	25–75%[c]	13%[d]

[a] Unknown or multiple methods
[b] Prescription fill records
[c] Electronic monitoring
[d] Pill count

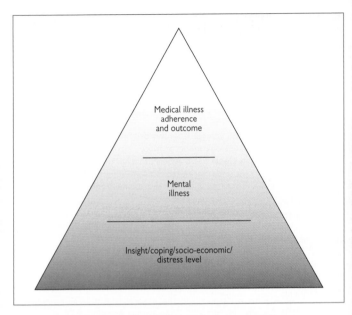

Figure 2.2 Role of psychiatric illness in disease adherence and outcome.

significant resistance to seeing a psychiatrist, long wait time before the appointment, and alcohol and drug problems predict whether a patient will miss the initial psychiatric appointment. Failure to attend follow-up appointments is associated with higher chance of hospitalization. People who miss their first psychiatric appointment after discharge have higher risk of re-admission. The nonadherence rate for follow-up appointments is 15% to 40%.[14]

Table 2.2 summarizes nonadherence rates for common psychiatric illnesses.

Schizophrenia

Despite the protective effect of antipsychotic adherence in schizophrenia[7] and clinicians' recommendations based on practice guidelines, patients often choose not to take antipsychotics. The rate of nonadherence is consistently found to be 30% to 60%.[15] Mojtabai and colleagues[16] showed that 63% of patients admitted for a first episode of schizophrenia stopped treatment with a first-generation antipsychotic within 1 year, with 51% of patients stopping their antipsychotic for longer than 30 days. Dolder and colleagues[17] showed that medication adherence was 50.1% for first-generation antipsychotics compared to 55% for second-generation oral antipsychotics for 12 months of treatment, as measured by prescription fill rates. In this study, patients on first-generation antipsychotics had an average of 7 days per month without medication versus 4 days per month for those on second-generation antipsychotics. Menzin and colleagues[18] obtained similar results, with 58% of patients on first-generation antipsychotics discontinuing medication over 1 year versus 33% of those on second-generation antipsychotics, based on paid prescription claims for California Medicaid recipients. In a review, Lacro and colleagues[15] found the nonadherence rate with first-generation long-acting antipsychotics to be as low as 4%, while in a retrospective study one third of

Table 2.2 Nonadherence Rate in Common Psychiatric Illnesses

	Schizo-phrenia[15, 17]	Major Depres-sion[23, 24, 25]	Bipolar Disorder[29, 39, 31]	Anxiety Disorders[32]	ADHD[34]	Alcohol Abuse and Depend-ence[36, 37]
Medication non adherence rate	30–60%[a]	51%[b]–69%[c]	21–50%[a,d]	57%[a]	26-48%[a]	35%[d]

[a] Unknown or multiple methods
[b] Prescription fill records
[c] Electronic monitoring
[d] Self-report

psychotic patients discontinued long-acting risperidone within 6 months; half were estimated to be partially nonadherent with injections.

The CATIE study[19] offered a broad view of antipsychotic drug treatment over a period of 18 months. In its first phase, the study compared perphenazine with second-generation antipsychotics (olanzapine, quetiapine, risperidone, and ziprasidone). While CATIE did not particularly address patient adherence to medication, the primary outcome measure was the discontinuation of treatment for any cause (including discontinuation as a shared decision made by the patient and doctors). In this $44 million study funded by the National Institute of Mental Health (NIMH), 74% of patients discontinued medication before 18 months (Fig. 2.3).

In phase II of the CATIE study, patients who joined the "efficacy pathway"[20] failed to respond to drugs they were assigned to in phase I and were randomly assigned either to the clozapine group or olanzapine, risperidone, or quetiapine group. Clozapine showed robust clinical effect and more patients stayed on it longer than for the other drugs (Fig. 2.4).

The phase II patients entering the "tolerability pathway"[21] were randomly assigned to double-blind treatment with ziprasidone, olanzapine, risperidone, or quetiapine (Fig. 2.5). The outcome measure here again was discontinuation for any reason, and the time to discontinuation was the same across all drugs, while discontinuation due to specific adverse effects differentiated the drugs used (weight gain was higher with olanzapine, there was no difference in QTc changes, there were increased prolactin levels with risperidone, cholesterol and triglyceride levels were increased with olanzapine and quetiapine and decreased with risperidone and ziprasidone).

As the figures show, the discontinuation rate was similarly high across phase I and both phase II pathways. The CATIE study acutely raised awareness about the limitations of our current treatment for schizophrenia, and the issue of antipsychotic adherence is even more important in the wake of its findings.

Mood disorders

"Depression hurts"

Depressed patients experience a high level of distress. Individuals rank depression as worse than other chronic diseases and are willing to pay significant amounts of money to eliminate depression; however, the side effects of medications can substantially reduce individuals' willingness to pay for depression treatment. In an interesting survey by Keith and Kane,[22] psychiatrists rated depression as a disease in which adherence was relatively easy to maintain to achieve a therapeutic effect (along the lines of rheumatoid arthritis or asthma), whereas weight reduction, schizophrenia, and exercise were rated as the conditions for which adherence is the most difficult to achieve. Despite this general belief, studies looking directly at

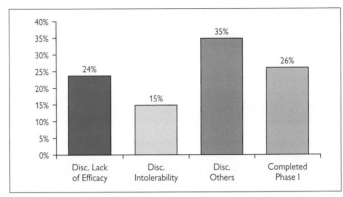

Figure 2.3 Antipsychotic discontinuation in phase I of the CATIE study[19].

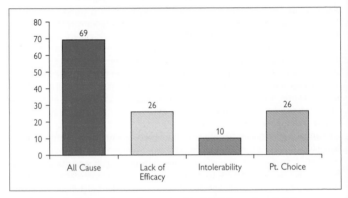

Figure 2.4 Antipsychotic discontinuation in phase II "efficacy pathway" of the CATIE study[20].

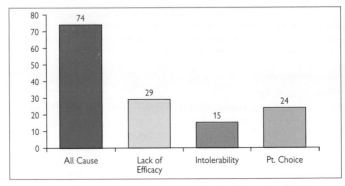

Figure 2.5 Antipsychotic discontinuation in phase II "tolerability pathway" of the CATIE study[21].

antidepressant treatment found significant nonadherence, with most depressed patients discontinuing their antidepressant in the first 6 months after their first prescription. A review of treatment adherence in unipolar depression literature published over a 25-year period found a median prevalence of nonadherence of 53%. Antidepressant treatment drop-out can be traced weekly as patients advance in treatment, with 30% of patients stopping these medications within 1 month and 45% to 60% by 3 months after initiation of treatment.[23] Patterns of nonadherence are similar for tricyclic antidepressants and serotonin reuptake inhibitors. Akincigil and colleagues,[24] using prescription fill records, found that in a large population of privately insured patients treated for a new episode of major depression, only 51% were adherent with antidepressants in the acute phase of illness and only 41.5% of those patients were adherent for the continuation phase (21% of patients remained adherent throughout both phases of treatment) (Fig. 2.6). Brown and colleagues[25] defined adherence to antidepressants measured with electronic bottle caps in a population of depressed patients in primary care as taking greater than 80% of prescribed doses. Adherence was found to be of 82% in the first month of treatment but declined to 69% at 3 months. The $35 million NIMH-funded 6-year Sequenced Treatment Alternatives to Relieve Depression (STAR*D) study used response and remission to antidepressants as outcome measures and like CATIE[19] did not specifically address antidepressant treatment adherence. However, the vast amount of data derived from STAR*D showed that our proficiency in helping depressed patients achieve response and remission decreases with treatment progression, with the number of people dropping out of treatment increasing with each stage (Table 2.3).[26]

This study clearly identified treatment intolerance as a major predictor for antidepressant treatment discontinuation; thus, the issue of antidepressant adherence comes into the spotlight again.

The Treatment for Adolescents with Depression Study (TADS) also showed a substantial level of treatment discontinuation. In the study, 439 depressed youths, ages 12 to 17 years, were randomly assigned to one of several groups: fluoxetine, cognitive–behavioral therapy (CBT), a combination of the two, or placebo pills.[27] After 12 weeks, 81.8% remained in the treatment group to which they were

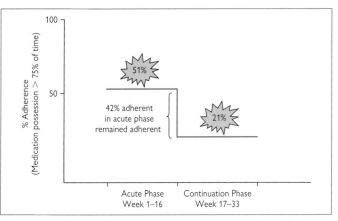

Figure 2.6 Adherence in acute and continuation treatment phases of major depressive disorder (based on data from Akincigil et al.[24])

Table 2.3 Treatment Outcomes and Dropout by Stage in STAR*D Study[26]

Stage	Remission	Response	Dropout for Any Reason Within 4 Weeks + Intolerable Adverse Effects*
1 (n = 3,671) Citalopram	36.8%	48.6%	16.3%
2 (n = 1,439) Bupropion or venlafaxine or sertraline or Citalopram + bupropion or + buspirone or + cognitive therapy or Cognitive therapy alone	30.6%	28.5%	19.5%
3 (n = 390) Level 2A: Bupropion or venlafaxine Level 3 Switch: Nortriptyline or mirtazapine or Augmentation: Lithium + bupropion or citalopram or sertraline or venlafaxine XR or Thyroid + bupropion or citalopram or sertraline or venlafaxine XR	13.7%	16.8%	25.6%
4 (n = 123) Level 3 Tranylcypromine or venlafaxine + mirtazapine	13.0%	16.3%	34.1%

assigned, without significant differences in discontinuation rates between treatment arms. During the first 12 weeks, Adjunct Services for Attrition Prevention (ASAP) was available to participants to address clinical crises (suicidality, self-harm) and dropout intentions. Two thirds of ASAP users either discontinued or modified treatment or dropped out prematurely. At the end of the 12-week acute phase, participants assigned to placebo were identified, dropped from the study, and treated. Three hundred twenty-seven patients remained randomized to one of the remaining three treatment conditions. By week 36, 25.7% of these participants exited the study due to consent withdrawal or loss to follow-up (19.6% in combination therapy, 29.4% in fluoxetine therapy, and 27.9% in CBT). Almost 50% of the 327 patients discontinued their originally randomized treatment, and the majority did so based on clinician recommendation. Here again, adherence was not specifically addressed.

Bipolar disorder

Scott and Pope[28] defined self-reported mood stabilizer partial adherence as having missed more than 30% of doses in the past month, based on sensitivity and specificity calculation. From their group of patients taking mood stabilizers, 32% were partially adherent according with this criterion, and over 60% of these subjects had subtherapeutic plasma levels of mood stabilizers. Risk factors for partial adherence were past history of nonadherence, denial of illness severity, and greater duration of treatment with a mood stabilizer as measured with the Lithium Attitudes Questionnaire (LAQ). The partially adherent groups of patients had more fear of medication side effects (rather than actually experiencing the side effects) and were more resistant to the idea of prophylaxis for mood disorders.

Rosa and colleagues,[29] using the same LAQ among other measurements, found that a low score on LAQ predicted adherence to lithium measured by plasma levels. They found that denial of illness and fear of side effects are common attitudes associated with nonadherence. Similarly, in a population of VA bipolar patients, greater insight into medication correlated with better adherence. Median long-term nonadherence with mood stabilizers is 41%, although there are overwhelming data to show that long-term adherence does in fact protect against recurrent mood episodes.[2,23]

DelBello and colleagues[30] measured outcome in adolescents with bipolar disorder for 1 year after their initial hospitalization for manic or mixed episode. Nonadherence was defined as having taken medication less than 25% of the time and partial adherence as having taken medication 25% to 75% of the time in the first year. Forty-two percent of adolescents were partially adherent and 23% were nonadherent. Predictors for nonadherence were comorbid ADHD, substance abuse, and lower socioeconomic status.

Strakowski and colleagues,[31] using DelBello's definition of adherence as reported by patients, families, and treating clinicians, presented data in two groups of adult patients, from Taiwan and the United States, followed for a year after their first manic or mixed episode. Seventy-nine percent of the patients from Taiwan and 50% of the patients from the United States were adherent with treatment. In this study, adherence correlated closely with outcome, as the U.S. patients spent much less time in remission from affective symptoms throughout the year after admission compared to Taiwanese patients (39% versus 79%).

Measurement of adherence, based on the medication possession ratio of lithium and anticonvulsants in a group of veterans, showed that only 54% of patients were fully adherent with medication (more than 80% medication possession). Younger age, being a member of an ethnic minority group, and presence of substance abuse were risks for nonadherence.

Over the short term (10 days), self-reported patient nonadherence with at least one dose of medication occurs in 33.8% of bipolar patients, while only 17.9% are recognized as nonadherent by their physicians.

Anxiety disorders

The National Epidemiologic Survey on Alcohol and Related Conditions (NESARC) found that anxiety disorders were present in 10% of people without a substance use disorder and 18% of people with substance use disorders. Fifty-seven percent of people with anxiety disorders are nonadherent with serotonin reuptake inhibitors and serotonin–norepinephrine reuptake inhibitors therapy at 6 months after initiation of their treatment, based on an 80% cutoff for their medication possession ratio; comorbidity with depression increases the likelihood of being adherent.

Toni and colleagues[32] designed a naturalistic 3-year follow-up study of patients with panic disorder with or without agoraphobia. Figure 2.7 shows the distribution of the 326 patients treated with antidepressants. Forty-eight patients dropped out and were untraceable. Of the remaining patients who interrupted their pharmacological treatment, most did so because of symptom remission after approximately 51 weeks of treatment.

Data about adherence in patients with obsessive-compulsive disorder (OCD) are scarce. In a study designed to validate an OCD Treatment Adherence Survey, 28% of patients reported nonadherence with CBT and 57% were nonadherent to psychotropic medications, assessed with the Adherence Determinants Questionnaire (ADQ).

ADHD

Medication compliance in the pediatric population averages 50% (as high as 85% to 95% for suburban immunizations to as low as 5% to 15% for urban adolescents). The adolescent age group carries the stereotype of "abusers of nonprescribed drugs" who are on the other hand "nonusers of prescribed drugs." Wolraich and colleagues,[33] in their adolescent ADHD review, emphasize the need to destigmatize the illness and ensure that adolescents and their families understand its neurobiological basis to overcome patients' negative attitudes and thus nonadherence. They cite the findings of a longitudinal 3-year study in which 48% of children between 9 and 15 years old stopped taking their medication, with the older children being more likely to stop medication.

Charach and colleagues[34] reported the adherence (defined as taking ADHD medication at least 5 days per week, measured with patient and parent reports) in a group of children with ADHD followed for 4 additional years after having completed a 12-month randomized controlled trial of methylphenidate and parent treatment programs. The adherence dropped from 53% in the second year to 36% at the completion of the fifth year of treatment. Patients who were adherent to stimulants showed greater improvement in teacher-reported symptoms over patients who were nonadherent or those who were not taking medications.

Patients with adult ADHD took a mean of 86.8% of their prescribed medication over the 2 weeks before the assessment of adherence. Patients with less than 80% medication adherence had significantly more severe ADHD symptoms.[35] Long-acting formulations of stimulants may improve adherence; an analysis of prescription fill records in more than 5,900 patients showed that fewer patients initiated on extended-release methylphenidate had 15- or 30-day gaps in ADHD therapy over 12 months compared with patients on immediate-release methylphenidate, and the duration of therapy was significantly longer for patients on the extended-release formulation.

Alcohol and substance abuse

The NESARC obtained valuable data on alcohol use from a sample of more than 4,000 individuals.[36] This retrospective study showed a significant level of recovery from alcohol dependence: 27% of people remitted, approximately 30% became asymptomatic or low-risk drinkers, 18% abstained from alcohol, and 25% remained dependent over the year preceding the interview. From the whole sample, only 25% of people sought treatment. Vaillant,[37] in a remarkable 60-year prospective study of inner-city men with alcohol abuse or dependence, found that 54% of men died by age 70, 12% were still abusing alcohol, 32% were abstinent, and 1% were controlled drinkers. Of the abstinent men in this cohort, only 36% attended Alcoholics Anonymous (AA). Of the minority of patients with alcohol use disorders who seek treatment, the available data on treatment adherence overwhelmingly come from studies comparing medication and psychosocial intervention strategies with medication alone or from comparisons between two medication groups.

In a study of alcohol dependence treatment for 12 weeks, Feeney and colleagues[38] found that patients receiving CBT and a combination of acamprosate

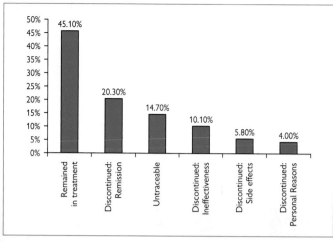

Figure 2.7 Adherence to antidepressants for panic disorder in a 3-year follow-up study[32].

and naltrexone had better adherence to treatment than the groups receiving CBT alone or CBT and either naltrexone or acamprosate; the group treated with CBT and medication combination had a better (although not statistically significant) abstinence outcome. Other studies of naltrexone treatment found adherence of 66% (defined as greater than 90% medication possession) in a 12-week rehabilitation program, whereas adherence with long-acting injections of naltrexone at 24 weeks was 61%.

Data about adherence to treatment for individual drug use disorders (which has an overall U.S. 12-month prevalence of 2%) is understandably scarce and usually reported as dropout rates in studies comparing medication interventions with psychotherapy or evaluating medication and psychotherapy together, similar to the findings for alcohol use disorders. One of the few pharmacological treatments for drug use disorders is for opiate dependence. Seventy-eight percent of patients with heroin dependence who entered a study of treatment with buprenorphine/naloxone stepped to methadone versus conventional methadone maintenance remained in treatment at 6 months.[39] Adherence to psychotherapy visits during 10 weeks of treatment with buprenorphine for patients dually diagnosed with opiate and cocaine dependence was 71%.

Interestingly, women are reported be heterogeneous in their rates of smoking cessation. Swan and colleagues[40] explored the possibility that genetic polymorphisms of dopamine receptor DRD2 gene explain this heterogeneity. The authors found association trends between the presence of at least one *A1* DRD2 allele in women and bupropion nonadherence related to side effects as well as a higher rate of smoking at 12 months of follow-up compared to women with two *A1* DRD2 alleles.

References

1. Kupfer DJ, Frank E, Perel JM, et al. Five-year outcome for maintenance therapies in recurrent depression. *Arch Gen Psychiatry.* 1992;49:769–773.

2. Gonzales-Pinto A, Mosquera F, Alonso M, et al. Suicidal risk in bipolar I disorder patients and adherence to long-term lithium treatment. *Bipolar Disord.* 2006;8:618–624.

3. Kane JM. Schizophrenia. *N Engl J Med.* 1996;334:34–41.

4. Robinson D, Woerner M, Alvir JM, et al. Predictors of relapse following response from a first episode of schizophrenia or schizoaffective disorder. *Arch Gen Psychiatry.* 1999;56:241–247.

5. Bangsberg DR, Hecht FM, Clague H, et al. Provider assessment of adherence to HIV Antiretroviral therapy. *J Acquir Immune Defic Syndr.* 2001;26:435–442.

6. Frishman WH. Importance of medication adherence in cardiovascular disease and the value of once-daily treatment regimens. *Cardiol Rev.* 2007;15:257–263.

7. Siegel D, Lopez J, Meier J. Antihypertensive medication adherence in the Department of Veterans Affairs. *Am J Med.* 2007;120:26–32.

8. Cramer JA. A systematic review of adherence with medications for diabetes. *Diabetes Care.* 2004;27:1218–1224.

9. Apter A, Reisine ST, Affleck G, Barrows E, Zuwallack R. Adherence with twice-daily dosing of inhaled steroids: socioeconomic and health belief differences. *Am J Respir Crit Care Med.* 1998;157:1810–1817.

10. Osterberg L, Blaschke T. Adherence to medication. *N Engl J Med.* 2005;353:487–497.

11. Glyngdal P, Sorensen P, Kistrup K. Non-compliance in community psychiatry: failed appointment in the referral system to psychiatric outpatient treatment. *Nord J Psychiatry.* 2002;56:151–156.

12. Livianos-Aldana L, Vila-Gomez M, Rojo-Moreno M, Luengo-Lopez MA. Patients who miss initial appointments in community psychiatry? A Spanish community analysis. *Int J Soc Psychiatry.* 1999;45:198–206.

13. Dotter JF, Labbate LA. Missed and canceled appointments at a military psychiatry clinic. *Mil Med.* 1998;163:58–60.

14. Mitchell AJ, Selmes T. A comparative survey of missed initial and follow-up appointments to psychiatric specialties in the United Kingdom. *Psychiatr Serv.* 2007;58:868–871.

15. Lacro JP, Dunn L, Dolder C, Leckband SG, Jeste DV. Prevalence and risk factors for medication non-adherence in patients with schizophrenia: a comprehensive review of recent literature. *J Clin Psychiatry.* 2002;63:892–909.

16. Mojtabai R, Lavelle J, Gibson PJ, et al. Gaps in use of antipsychotics after discharge by first admission patients with schizophrenia, 1989 to 1996. *Psychiatr Serv.* 2002;53:337–339.

17. Dolder C, Lacro JP, Dunn L, Jeste DV. Antipsychotic medication adherence: is there a difference between typical and atypical agents? *Am J Psychiatry.* 2002;159:103–108.

18. Menzin J, Boulanger L, Friedman M, Mackell J, Lloyd JR. Treatment adherence associated with conventional and atypical antipsychotics in a large state Medicaid program. *Psychiatr Serv.* 2003;54:719–723.

19. Lieberman JA, Stroup TS, McEvoy JP, et al. Effectiveness of antipsychotic drugs in patients with chronic schizophrenia. *N Engl J Med.* 2005;353:1209–1223.

20. McEvoy JP, Lieberman JA, Stroup TS, et al. Effectiveness of clozapine versus olanzapine, quetiapine, and risperidone in patients with chronic schizophrenia who did not respond to prior antipsychotic treatment. *Am J Psychiatry.* 2006;163:600–610.

21. Stroup TS, Lieberman JA, McEvoy JP, et al. Effectiveness of olanzapine, quetiapine, risperidone and ziprasidone in patients with chronic schizophrenia following discontinuation of a previous atypical antipsychotic. Am J Psychiatry. 2006;163:611–622.

22. Keith SJ, Kane JM. Partial compliance and patient consequences in schizophrenia: our patients can do better. J Clin Psychiatry 2003;64:1308–1315.

23. Lingam R, Scott J. Treatment non-adherence in affective disorders. Acta Psychiatr Scand. 2002;105:164–172.

24. Akincigil A, Bowblis J, Levin C, et al. Adherence to antidepressant treatment among privately insured patients diagnosed with depression. Med Care. 2007; 45:363–369.

25. Brown C, Battista DR, Sereika S, Bruehlman RD, Dunbar-Jacob J, Thase ME. How can you improve antidepressant adherence? J Fam Practice. 2007;56:356–363.

26. Rush AJ, Trivedi MH, Wisniewski SR, et al. Acute and long-term outcomes in depressed outpatients requiring one or several treatment steps: a STAR*D report. Am J Psychiatry. 2006;163:1906–1917.

27. Emslie G, Kratochvil C, Vitiello B, et al. Treatment for Adolescents with Depression Study (TADS): safety results. J Am Acad Child Adolesc Psychiatry. 2006;45:1440–1455.

28. Scott J, Pope M. Non-adherence with mood stabilizers: prevalence and predictors. J Clin Psychiatry. 2002;63:384–390.

29. Rosa AR, Marco M, Fachel JM, Kapczinski F, Stein AT, Barros HM. Correlation between drug treatment adherence and lithium treatment attitudes and knowledge by bipolar patients. Prog Neuropsychopharmacol Biol Psychiatry. 2007;31:217–224.

30. DelBello M, Hanserman D, Adler CM, Fleck DE, Strakowski SM. Twelve-month outcome of adolescents with bipolar disorder following first hospitalization for a manic or mixed episode. Am J Psychiatry. 2007;164:582–590.

31. Strakowski SM, Tsai SY, DelBello MP, et al. Outcome following a first manic episode: cross-national U.S. and Taiwan comparison. Bipolar Disord. 2007;9:820–827.

32. Toni C, Perugi G, Frare F, Mata B, Akiskal HS. Spontaneous treatment discontinuation in panic disorder patients treated with antidepressants. Acta Psychiatr Scand. 2004;110:130–137.

33. Wolraich ML, Wibbelsman CJ, Brown TE, et al. Attention-deficit/hyperactivity disorder among adolescents: a review of diagnosis, treatment and clinical implications. Pediatrics. 2005;115:1734–1746.

34. Carach A, Ickowicz A, Schachar R. Stimulant treatment over five years: adherence, effectiveness and adverse effects. J Am Acad Child Adolesc Psychiatry. 2004; 43:559–566.

35. Safren SA, Duran P, Yovel I, Perlman C, Sprich S. Medication adherence in psychopharmacologically treated adults with ADHD. J Attent Disord. 2007; 10:257–260.

36. Dawson DA, Grant BF, Stinson F, et al. Recovery from DSM-IV alcohol dependence: United States, 2001–2002. Addiction. 2005;100:281–292.

37. Vaillant GE. A 60-year follow-up of alcoholic men. Addiction. 2003; 98:1043–1051.

38. Feeney GFX, Connor JP, Young R, Tucker J, McPherson A. Combined acamprosate and naltrexone, with cognitive behavioural therapy is superior to either

medication alone for alcohol abstinence: a single centre's experience with pharmacotherapy. *Alcohol Alcoholism*. 2006;41:321–327.

39. Kakko J, Gronbladh L, Svanborg KD, et al. A stepped care strategy using buprenorphine and methadone versus conventional methadone maintenance in heroin dependence: a randomized controlled trial. *Am J Psychiatry*. 2007;164:797–803.

40. Swan GE, Valdes AM, Ring HZ, et al. Dopamine receptor DRD2 genotype and smoking cessation outcome following treatment with bupropion SR. *Pharmacogenomics J*. 2005;5:21–29.

Chapter 3

Reasons for medication nonadherence

As has been stated before, there are multiple and varied reasons why a person chooses not to take medications. Often we consider this within a "disease-specific" framework—for instance, people with schizophrenia do not take medicines because they lack insight, depressed patients stop medicines due to side effects. However, perhaps the most salient feature of medication adherence is simply the usual adage that every patient is different. The patient may stop medications for any number of reasons, and it is our responsibility to try to understand the individual circumstances for that patient. Some reasons why patients do not take medications are listed in Figure 3.1.

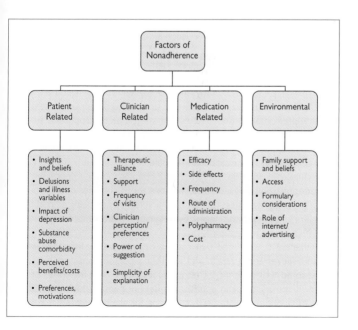

Figure 3.1 Factors associated with nonadherence to medication.

Patient-related factors

Lack of insight is the major reason, irrespective of type of mental illness, why people do not adhere to treatment. In a study of compliance to therapy in schizophrenia, O'Donnell and colleagues[1] found that lack of insight was one of the strongest predictors of whether the patients took their medicine. Lack of awareness of illness may cause a patient to feel as if he or she is being forced by others to undergo unnecessary treatment. Insight is itself a complex phenomenon and is not simply an "all-or-none" state. Amador and Gorman[2] have described specific components of insight, including awareness of present illness, awareness of signs and symptoms related to illness, attribution of current signs and symptoms to the illness, and understanding of the usefulness of treatment. It is also important to distinguish current insight from retrospective insight. Amador's studies have shown that almost 60% of patients with schizophrenia have substantial lack of awareness of their condition.[2] Many patients are also unaware of the presence of related symptoms.

Growing research suggests a potential neurobiological component to impaired insight in schizophrenia, although findings have not been consistent. In a meta-analysis of 35 neuropsychological studies involving over 2,000 patients, Aleman and colleagues[3] found a significant positive relationship between insight and general cognitive functioning. Several researchers have also shown a more specific association between insight and frontal lobe function. In a study involving 108 schizophrenic patients from three different countries, Young and colleagues[4] found a consistent association between poor scores on the Wisconsin Card Sorting Test (WCST), a measure of executive function, and lack of awareness of illness. In a 2006 review article, Shad and colleagues[5] highlighted a large number of studies reporting a relationship between insight deficits and impaired cognitive performance, particularly on measures of frontal lobe function such as the WCST. Shad and colleagues[6] have also documented decreased right dorsolateral prefrontal cortex volumes in first-episode schizophrenia patients with poor insight compared to those with good insight.

Of course, patient-related factors affecting adherence are made all the more complex by whatever beliefs the patient holds about his or her illness. For example, in addition to limited understanding among depressed men about depression being a disease, men are apt to consider depression as a sign of personal weakness, of lack of character, of not being a "real man." The NIMH addressed this stigma by designing a national campaign entitled "Real Men, Real Depression."[7]

In Chapter 1, we noted that culture can powerfully influence what a person believes about health and whether a person considers himself or herself to be ill or suffering from a particular illness. The high rates of alcoholism in some European countries reflect not only a higher per capita intake of alcohol but also a high tolerance for alcohol-related disruptions such that people can have advanced alcohol dependency before they realize they have become an alcoholic.

Distinct symptoms of the illness may lead to medication nonadherence. For example, anticholinesterases are often given to people with mild cognitive impairment or early dementia, but these patients may forget to take their medicines. People with schizophrenia may believe they are being poisoned and, thus, refuse to take any medications. Adolescents with ADHD may be inattentive and not organized enough in the mornings to remember to take their medications. The depressed patient may be withdrawn, apathetic, and forgetful about taking medication. The list goes on. It is important to consider the interaction between illness/symptoms and medication nonadherence, particularly as it might influence the selection and formulation of subsequent medication treatments. In general, there is a positive relationship between severity of illness and medication nonadherence (Fig. 3.2).[8] Again, this is most obvious in dementia, but it is also common in schizophrenia and mood disorders. It is, of course, hard to know which came first: is the nonadherence because the illness is so bad that it impedes the process of medication adherence, or is the illness severe in the absence of treatment due to medication nonadherence?

Comorbidity of alcohol or substance abuse is a strong predictor of medication nonadherence,[9] and this comorbidity is common: it is estimated that 70% to 80% of patients with bipolar disorder abuse alcohol or drugs at some time during their illness. The figures for schizophrenia range from 40% to 60%. Although this is sometimes not considered, there is also surreptitious abuse of alcohol or drugs among the elderly. Although it is sometimes cited that patients simply are being careful in following their doctor's advice not to mix medicines and alcohol, invariably the relationship is much more complex. Dual-diagnosis patients are notoriously poor at adhering to their prescribed medications. This is complicated by homelessness, by lack of support, by a culture that promotes drug use but not adherence to prescribed medications, by medical problems, by severity of illness, and by lack of money. Also, these patients may have an even greater propensity to side effects of medications.

One of the main reasons why delusional disorder is so debilitating is that invariably patients either do not commence medications or do not

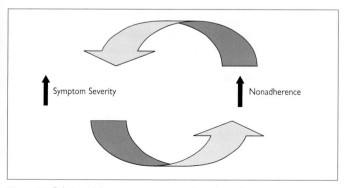

Figure 3.2 Relationship between symptom severity and nonadherence.

adhere to them.[10] They simply do not believe they are ill, and since their delusional system is so firm and encapsulated, trying to convince them otherwise tends to be futile. They have so many aspects of their life where they are "normal" that getting them to see that that their delusional behavior is abnormal and warrants medication treatment is a real challenge. For these patients, it is not so much their cultural experience or environment that shapes their beliefs; they simply assert, "I'm not sick. I don't need medications."

Clinician-related factors

The quality of the relationship between the patient and doctor is another powerful determinant of medication nonadherence. Patients who feel their doctor understands their situation, communicates effectively with them, and has their best interest at heart are much more likely to adhere to prescribed medication. Conversely, patients who are distrustful of their physician or are uncertain about his or her competency are less likely to take their prescribed medications. Although it seems just too obvious to be worth mentioning, patients who are paranoid and have specific delusions about their doctor are notoriously nonadherent with medications.

Frank and Gunderson[11] showed that the quality of the patient–physician relationship predicted subsequent medication adherence. Following a 2-year study on psychotherapy in schizophrenic patients during which more than half of the participants dropped out of treatment, Frank and Gunderson decided to retrospectively examine the impact of therapeutic alliance. Though less than 30% of participants had developed good alliances with their physicians within the first 6 months of the study, those who did were less likely to quit psychotherapy, were more likely to comply with prescribed medication regimens, and showed greater overall improvement in symptoms using less medication than participants with weaker alliances.[11]

A recent study of patients with bipolar I disorder receiving pharmacotherapy over a 28-month period also showed a positive effect of working alliance on the number of months that participants remained in treatment.[12] There is also some evidence that how the physician proposes and describes a medication choice affects the patient's decision about taking that medication. If the physician is concerned about side effects, this will pass directly onto the patient. For example, the use of clozapine remains low despite its proven effectiveness over other medications for patients with severe schizophrenia. One reason contributing to this low use is the fear among doctors that the drug has too many side effects and that monitoring for agranulocytosis is overly burdensome.[13] Conversely, if a doctor "really believes" in a medication, this is likely to prompt the patient to remain longer on this medication.

The frequency of clinic visits is probably also a contributor to medication adherence, as patients who are more closely monitored are more likely to remain on their prescribed medications. Systems of care where access to the physician is limited or delayed may contribute to medication nonadherence. It is certainly common for patients to state that they stopped their medication because "I couldn't get my prescription refilled," "I couldn't get an appointment with the doctor," "the doctor wasn't able to see me for 6 weeks." The extent to which missed appointments by patients is a symptom or a cause of medication nonadherence can be difficult to determine; often, both aspects are in play.

The use of alternative medications is a less appreciated aspect of this issue. According to the National Center for Complementary and Alternative Medicine, a survey distributed to over 30,000 adults in the United States showed that 36% used some form of complementary and alternative medicine (CAM) in 2002. If the definition of CAM is expanded to include health-related prayer and megavitamin therapy, the number rises to 62%. The majority of those surveyed reported using CAM as an adjunct to as opposed to a substitute for conventional treatment.[14] CAM use will be discussed further in Chapter 6.

Medication-related factors

Side effects are a powerful reason for people to stop taking their medications. In a recent survey conducted by Mental Health America, 69% of people with schizophrenia reported that they had discontinued use of medication due to side effects that had a negative impacted on their quality of life.[15] Patients may often not fill a prescription or stop taking a medication because they fear some serious side effect. In bipolar disorder, patients can become nonadherent precisely because of the effectiveness of the medication in controlling their symptoms: they miss the highs of bipolar mania. Many patients dislike the idea of medication controlling their mood, and others dislike taking medication because it reminds them that they have a chronic mental illness.[16] The patient's beliefs about the illness may also contribute to stopping treatment prematurely. This is particularly evident in depression. It has been shown that a patient's perceptions of the stigma associated with depression at the start of treatment will predict subsequent medication adherence.[17]

One example is a patient who does not even start an antipsychotic medication because he has read that it could cause neuroleptic malignant syndrome and "I'm not going to risk it." However, it is more often the case that less radically serious side effects result in medication nonadherence (Fig. 3.3). This is both because they are more common and because they are tolerated less by patients.[18] Somnolence is a good example. While somnolence can certainly be associated with risk (e.g., being sleepy while driving, falling asleep while the kitchen stove is on), in general this is more of a burdensome side effect than one that is medically serious. It is, however, a very common reason why people stop their medication. They dislike feeling sleepy or "drugged-up." They cannot do daily tasks and feel very frustrated by this. They may have to go back to bed during the day because of sedative side effects. They may not be able to read, to travel, or to meet friends because they are "too tired" on their medication.

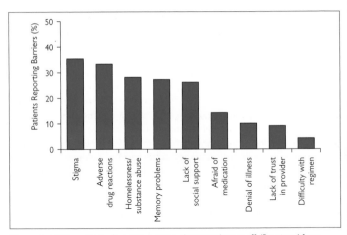

Figure 3.4 Why patients discontinue antipsychotic medications.[22] (Reprinted from Hudson TJ, Owen RR, Thrush CR, et al. A pilot study of barriers to medication adherence in schizophrenia. *Journal of Clinical Psychiatry*, Vol. 65; 211–6, © 2004, with permission from Physicians Postgraduate Press.)

Friends and family members may (rightly) reinforce these negative experiences by pointing out that they appear "drugged-up" or "spacey" and should not drive because they are oversedated. Indeed, oversedation evokes powerful negative responses from family members. They want their loved one to be less anxious, calmer, and able to function, but they do not want him or her to be "drugged-up." Family members are very intolerant of this effect. Thus, one can appreciate the significance of sedation as a side effect. In terms of medication nonadherence, it is one of the worst side effects for a therapeutic agent to have.

Sexual side effects are also very poorly tolerated and lead quickly to nonadherence. This is particularly so in depression. A 2002 review article by Gregorian and colleagues found that 30% to 60% of SSRI-treated patients may experience some form of treatment-induced sexual dysfunction.[19]

Other adverse effects that lead quickly to medication nonadherence include motor restlessness (akathisia), nausea and vomiting, and tremor or gait unsteadiness. Although certain patients are more likely to get side effects (e.g., constipation from medications is much more likely to occur among elderly patients), it is also important to appreciate that patients vary widely in their tolerance of any given side effect. For example, weight gain is a common side effect of many psychotropic medications. This adverse effect is far better tolerated by a 35-year-old man who is already overweight than it is by a 26-year-old slim woman. In addition, a 26-year-old slim woman who has always been weight-conscious is far less likely to be adherent to a medication that is causing weight gain than another 26-year-old slim woman who is less focused on weight (and in fact stays thin not through diet but exercises also). The context of the side effect matters greatly.

Other side effects may be surprisingly well tolerated. For example, one would consider that drooling at night (a common side effect of clozapine therapy) would be a frequent reason for stopping this medication,[18] but surprisingly patients seem to tolerate this side effect well. Tardive dyskinesia is a serious side effect and may be a reason for the patient not even to try a medication. However, some patients do not even recognize when they have these abnormal involuntary movements: in one study, 46.5% of patients were at least moderately unaware these movements.[20]

It is the perceived impact of the side effect that matters most. In other words, when it comes to a side effect, it's what the person thinks is happening rather than the prevailing medical circumstances. For example, a depressed man tries an antidepressant medication for 5 days and then stops. At the return clinic visit he says he stopped the medication because "it made my depression worse." The drug is not likely to worsen depression directly; it is more likely that the person's depression deteriorated further for some other, unrelated reason. On the other hand, the patient who says that the medication "made my depression worse" may be experiencing more fatigue (possibly medication-related). Sometimes a patient with schizophrenia may refuse to take his or her antipsychotic medication because he or she feels "it makes the voices worse." Again, this is implausible. This is one reason why it is so important to ensure that patients and their loved ones are educated about what medicines can, and cannot, do. A study by Bull and colleagues[21] involving 401 depressed patients being treated with SSRIs showed that effective communication about adverse drug effects significantly reduced the likelihood of treatment discontinuation. In addition, patients who discussed adverse events with physicians were over five times more likely to switch medication. Switching medications may result in more favorable outcomes, since a patient who is intolerant to one antidepressant may not be affected the same way by another.

Efficacy, dosage, and route of administration

Even more so than because of adverse effects, patients stop medications due to lack of efficacy of the drug: people will not continue to take a treatment they do not consider is helping them. This is a complex issue because we know there is wide interindividual variation in medications. It is a fundamental weakness of our current treatment paradigm that both treatment response and tolerability to any given medication vary greatly from patient to patient. Patients decide to discontinue medications for many different reasons (Figs. 3.3, 3.4, 3.5).[22-24]

This inherent variability underlies our current inability to predict how an individual patient may respond to the selected medication. This uncertainty undermines the treatment expectations and promotes frequent switching of medications in search of the "right fit." Taking psychotropic medications is not like taking an antibiotic: with an antibiotic, the patient knows the right dose and can expect to feel better within 3 to 5 days, and the drug works for most people. In that situation, the likelihood of medication adherence

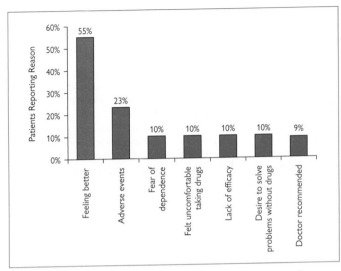

Figure 3.4 Patient-reported reasons for nonadherence with antidepressants.[23]

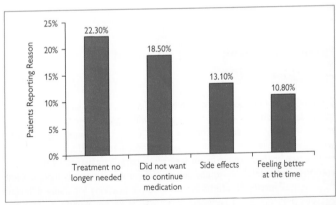

Figure 3.5 Patient-reported reasons for discontinuing treatment for bipolar disorder.[24]

is raised by the expectation of success of the treatment. It is simply not so for treatment with psychotropic medications.

The dosage of the medication also contributes to the potential for medication nonadherence. Too low a dose (i.e., a dose that is subtherapeutic) invites nonadherence because the patient ends up taking a medication that will not work for him or her. A dose that falls within the therapeutic range may work, but here again there is wide variation. For instance, it has been found that the higher the blood level of valproic acid while still within its range (50 to 100 mg/mL), the more likely it is that the patient with bipolar symptoms will respond.[25] On the other hand, many side effects are dose-dependent—that is, the higher the dose, the greater the likelihood that the side effect will occur. Also, the more medication taken, the more severe the side effect will be. It is thus a fine balancing act to find the right dose for the right patient. This is one reason why pharmacogenetics holds promise, as will be discussed further in Chapter 5.

It seems intuitive that the route of administration would affect medication adherence. However, surprisingly, this has not been as clearly established as one might anticipate. For example, it seems intuitive that dissolvable, "melt-in-your-mouth" tablet wafers would improve medication adherence over oral tablets. This has not been proven. Similarly, long-acting injections should be associated with enhanced adherence. However, in a study by Buchanan and colleagues,[26] there was no difference in treatment adherence over 2 years of care in patients taking either oral or injectable antipsychotic medications. Indeed, while depot antipsychotic preparations are proposed for patients with adherence problems, the effect of this strategy may be mostly through the elimination of covert medication nonadherence—that is, if the patient does not show up for the injection, the clinic becomes aware of his or her nonadherence.

Both the complexity of the medication regimen and polypharmacy heighten the risk of nonadherence. Medications that need to be taken several times a day are associated with a greater likelihood of partial or complete nonadherence. Indeed, there have been efforts to minimize this effect, such as the development of longer-lasting forms. Examples include the once-weekly tablet of fluoxetine and extended-release forms of antidepressants and anticonvulsants. These will be discussed further in Chapter 5.

Environmental factors

The support and involvement of family members is a powerful predictor of whether a patient will take a prescribed medication.[1] Financial burden is another major reason why people do not take medications. Patients may be unable to afford medication because their health insurance does not cover the entire amount of the medication, the medication is not on the insurance company's formulary (in which case the patient may be liable for the full cost of the drug), or the patient does not have any insurance. The National Mental Health Association has an important policy document entitled "Pennywise & Pound Foolish: Restricting Access to Psychotropic Medications" that addresses this complex topic in great detail.[27] NAMI and the Depression Bipolar Support Alliance (DBSA) are also strong proponents for full access to psychotropic medications.[28,29]

These difficulties are compounded by differences in health insurance coverage and medication availability between inpatient and outpatient treatment settings. In general, inpatient settings are more inclusive of medication choices and insurance coverage is less of an immediate concern. However, all too often the patient may be started on a medication as an inpatient only to find out upon discharge that his or her insurance plan does not cover this medication. This can directly lead to nonadherence or it can lead to a (rapid) switching of medications to remedy this situation. This switching of medications can later result in nonadherence. Conversely, a patient who is hospitalized might not be able to get access to a regularly prescribed medication because this medication is not on the hospital's formulary. In this instance, the patient is usually offered a substitution medication, one of a similar drug class.

The extent to which formulary processes, drug-review procedures, and medication authorization procedures contribute to nonadherence is likely to be significant but has not been quantified. Delays in authorization of a medication or denial of that medication choice would intuitively undermine medication adherence. The extent to which preferred choice strategies add to medication nonadherence is another important yet poorly understood consideration. Preferred choice strategies are typically implemented to cut down on the medication costs to large organizations that manage their formulary.

One measure being used by Medicaid to control rising drug costs is the implementation of prior authorization policies, which require that specific conditions be met before drug reimbursement is provided. As of March 2006, over 40% of state Medicaid programs had prior authorization policies concerning atypical antipsychotics.[30] Soumerai and colleagues[31] studied the effect of Maine's prior authorization policy on atypical antipsychotic use from July 2003 to February 2004. They found that patients who initiated treatment with atypical antipsychotics while the policy was in effect had a 29% greater risk of treatment discontinuity than patients who began treatment before the policy took effect. Discontinuity was defined as a gap in therapy of 30 or more days or switching to or augmentation with another antipsychotic. In comparison, there was no change in discontinuity rates in New Hampshire, a state that did not have a prior authorization policy for atypical antipsychotics during that time. Parenthetically, if these policies inadvertently contribute to medication nonadherence, then the cost of care is far more likely to be more expensive, since nonadherence is often a harbinger for relapse of illness and subsequent hospitalization.

The impact of formularies and prescription drug plans on medication adherence is being examined closely. After the implementation of Medicare prescription drug benefits (Medicare Part D) in 2006, a large national survey of psychiatrists reported high rates of access problems and medication discontinuation among dual-eligible psychiatric patients (whose prescription coverage changed from Medicaid to Medicare Part D).[32] Results of the survey indicated that during the first 4 months of Part D implementation, over half of patients covered had experienced one or more problems with medication access or continuity. Over 20% were reported to have discontinued medication due to drug plan administrative issues, changes in coverage, management of benefits, or copayments. Nearly 20% had to switch to a new medication despite clinical stability taking another. In this sense, patients may be unable to maintain adherence even if they desire to, thus increasing the risk of a poor clinical outcome.[32]

Medication nonadherence in children and the elderly

The majority of the factors related to medication nonadherence described above also apply to the distinct population of children who take psychotropic medication, as well as to geriatric patients. However, some additional comments are relevant in each circumstance.

Among children, the impact of relatives or caregivers on medication adherence is substantial. Children often cannot appreciate the seriousness of their illness and are often ill equipped to evaluate the risk–benefit profile of a given drug. Therefore, the role of the caregiver becomes an important factor in a child's adherence to medication. For example, a significant relationship between pediatric nonadherence and poor parent–child communication, high caregiver stress, poor caregiver quality of life, and poor caregiver cognitive function has been shown in children infected with HIV.[33] It is important for the physician to establish a good relationship with both the child and the parent or caregiver while fostering understanding of both parties concerning the importance of following prescribed treatment plans. In one study of children prescribed oral antibiotics, adherence increased by 22% when patients and their caregivers were given written instructions plus counseling on the importance of taking the medication.[34]

Of course, even if a child does not understand the importance of medication for a given illness, he or she still may experience side effects. As a result, children may be more prone to discontinue medication use. Several studies have shown that medication adverse effects and palatability factors can contribute to pediatric nonadherence.[35] Therefore, the importance of vigilance by family members cannot be overstated. It has been shown that efforts to regularize the time that a child takes medications daily can be particularly important. Simpler schedules and treatment regimens have been shown to enhance compliance in children.[35]

In the elderly, the impact of cognitive impairment can be substantial.[36] Simple forgetting can easily undermine treatment. The elderly have also been shown to have poorer functional health literacy, defined as the ability to read, understand, and act on health information such as prescription labels and instructions.[37] Other factors that may place the elderly at increased risk of nonadherence include diminished visual acuity, hearing, and manual dexterity. This may make reading medication labels, differentiating pill colors, and opening prescription bottles more of a challenge in older patients.[38] Geriatric patients commonly take multiple medications, which may complicate adherence, although some studies have shown the opposite to be true.[38]

References

1. O'Donnell C, Donohoe G, Sharkey L, et al. Compliance therapy: a randomised controlled trial in schizophrenia. *BMJ.* 2003;327:834.

2. Amador XF, Gorman JM. Psychopathologic domains and insight in schizophrenia. *Psychiatr Clin North Am.* 1998;21:27–42.

3. Aleman A, Agrawal N, Morgan KD, David AS. Insight in psychosis and neuropsychological function: meta-analysis. *Br J Psychiatry.* 2006;189:204–212.

4. Young DA, Zakzanis KK, Bailey C, et al. Further parameters of insight and neuropsychological deficit in schizophrenia and other chronic mental disease. *J Nerv Ment Dis.* 1998;186:44–50.

5. Shad MU, Tamminga CA, Cullum M, Haas GL, Keshavan MS. Insight and frontal cortical function in schizophrenia: a review. *Schizophr Res.* 2006;86:54–70.

6. Shad MU, Muddasani S, Prasad K, Sweeney JA, Keshavan MS. Insight and prefrontal cortex in first-episode schizophrenia. *Neuroimage.* 2004;22:1315–1320.

7. National Institute of Mental Health. *Real Men, Real Depression.* http://www.nimh.nih.gov/health/publications/real-men-real-depression.pdf. Accessed August 10, 2008.

8. Ascher-Svanum H, Zhu B, Faries D, Lacro JP, Dolder CR. A prospective study of risk factors for nonadherence with antipsychotic medication in the treatment of schizophrenia. *J Clin Psychiatry.* 2006;67:1114–1123.

9. Buckley PF. Prevalence and consequences of the dual diagnosis of substance abuse and severe mental illness. *J Clin Psychiatry.* 2006;67:5–9.

10. Smith DA, Buckley PF. Pharmacotherapy of delusional disorders in the context of offending and the potential for compulsory treatment. *Behav Sci Law.* 2006;24:351–367.

11. Frank AF, Gunderson JG. The role of the therapeutic alliance in the treatment of schizophrenia. Relationship to course and outcome. *Arch Gen Psychiatry.* 1990;47:228–236.

12. Gaudiano BA. Miller IW. Patients' expectancies, the alliance in pharmacotherapy, and treatment outcomes in bipolar disorder. *J Consult Clin Psychol.* 2006;74:671–676.

13. Moore TA, Buchanan RW, Buckley PF, et al. The Texas Medication Algorithm Project antipsychotic algorithm for schizophrenia: 2006 update. *J Clin Psychiatry.* 2007;68:1751–1762.

14. Barnes P, Powell-Griner E, McFann K, Nahin R. *Complementary and Alternative Medicine Use Among Adults: United States, 2002. CDC Advance Data Report #343:* May 27, 2004.

15. Mental Health America. *Communicating About Health: A Mental Health America Survey of People with Schizophrenia and Providers.* Http://www.nmha.org/go/surveys. Accessed July 9, 2008.

16. Lingam R, Scott J. Treatment non-adherence in affective disorders. *Acta Psychiatr Scand.* 2002;105:164–172.

17. Sirey JA, Bruce ML, Alexopoulos GS, et al. Perceived stigma as a predictor of treatment discontinuation in young and older outpatients with depression. *Am J Psychiatry.* 2001;158:479–481.

18. Miller DD. Review and management of clozapine side effects. *J Clin Psychiatry.* 2000;61:14–17.

19. Gregorian RS, Golden KA, Bahce A, Goodman C, Kwong WJ, Khan ZM. Antidepressant-induced sexual dysfunction. *Ann Pharmacother.* 2002; 36:1577–1589.

20. Arango C, Adami H, Sherr JD, Thaker GK, Carpenter WT. Relationship of awareness of dyskinesia in schizophrenia to insight into mental illness. *Am J Psychiatry.* 1999;156:1097–1099.

21. Bull SA, Hu XH, Hunkeler EM, et al. Discontinuation of use and switching of antidepressants: influence of patient-physician communication. *JAMA.* 2002;288:1403–1409.

22. Hudson TJ, Owen RR, Thrush CR, et al. A pilot study of barriers to medication adherence in schizophrenia. *J Clin Psychiatry.* 2004;65:211–216.

23. Demyttenaere K, Enzlin P, Dewe W, et al. Compliance with antidepressants in a primary care setting, 1: Beyond lack of efficacy and adverse events. *J Clin Psychiatry.* 2001;62:30–33.

24. Baldessarini RJ, Perry R, Pike J. Factors associated with treatment nonadherence among US bipolar disorder patients. *Hum Psychopharmacol.* 2008;23:95–105.

25. Allen MH, Hirschfeld RM, Wozniak PJ, Baker JD, Bowden CL. Linear relationship of valproate serum concentration to response and optimal serum levels for acute mania. *Am J Psychiatry.* 2006;163:272–275.

26. Buchanan RW, Kirkpatrick B, Summerfelt A, Hanlon TE, Levine J, Carpenter WR Jr. Clinical predictors of relapse following neuroleptic withdrawal. *Biol Psychiatry.* 1992;32:72–78.

27. National Mental Health Association. http://www.nmha.org. Accessed August 2, 2008.

28. National Alliance on Mental Illness. http://www.nami.org. Accessed August 2, 2008.

29. Depression Bipolar Support Alliance. http://www.dbsalliance.org. Accessed August 2, 2008.

30. Polinski JM, Wang PS, Fischer MA. Medicaid's prior authorization program and access to atypical antipsychotic medications. *Health Aff.* 2007;26:750–760.

31. Soumerai S, Zhang F, Ross-Degnan D, et al. Use of atypical antipsychotic drugs for schizophrenia in Maine Medicaid following a policy change. *Health Aff.* 2008; 27:185–195.

32. West JC, Wilk JE, Muszynski IL, et al. Medication access and continuity: the experiences of dual-eligible psychiatric patients during the first 4 months of the Medicare prescription drug benefit. *Am J Psychiatry.* 2007;164:789–796.

33. Mellins CA, Brackis-Cott E, Dolezal C, Abrams EJ. The role of psychosocial and family factors in adherence to antiretroviral treatment in human immunodeficiency virus-infected children. *Pediatr Infect Dis J.* 2004;23:1035–1041.

34. Colcher IS, Bass JW. Penicillin treatment of streptococcal pharyngitis. A comparison of schedules and the role of specific counseling. *JAMA.* 1972; 222:657–659.

35. Winnick S, Lucas DO, Hartman AL, Toll D. How do you improve compliance? *Pediatrics.* 2005;115:718–724.

36. Ruscin JM, Semla TP. Assessment of medication management skills in older outpatients. *Ann Pharmacother.* 1996;30:1083–1088.

37. Baker DW, Gazmararian JA, Sudano J, Patterson M. The association between age and health literacy among elderly persons. *J Gerontol B Psychol Sci Soc Sci.* 2000;55:S368–374.

38. MacLaughlin EJ, Raehl C, Treadway AK, Sterling TL, Zoller DP, Bond CA. Assessing medication adherence in the elderly: Which tools to use in clinical practice? *Drugs Aging.* 2005;22:231–255.

Chapter 4

Detection and monitoring of nonadherence

Since the time of Hippocrates, adherence to treatment has been recognized as a critical factor in treating all illnesses, medical and psychiatric.[1] Medication adherence is related to clinical outcome, and suboptimal adherence reduces the effectiveness of a treatment intervention. Simply put, no medication will be successful in treating an illness if the medication itself is not taken as prescribed.

> "All the medicines in the world are for naught if we cannot get people to take them."

—*C. Everett Koop*

Knowing the extent to which a patient is adherent to his or her medication regimen is paramount in clinical practice. Clinicians tend to have inaccurate estimates of their patients' adherence rates to medications, and often clinicians want to believe that their patients are 100% adherent.[1] The reality is, however, that patients may take very little of their prescribed medications or sometimes take more than what has been prescribed. Velligan and colleagues[2] showed considerable disagreement between physician impression of adherence to antipsychotics compared with pill count and electronic monitoring. "Knowing" is one thing, and knowing *with a degree of certainty* is another. Relying solely on a clinician's thoughts on level of adherence is not accurate or adequate. While detecting and monitoring adherence is not easy, routine measuring of adherence through direct or indirect methods is a necessary component of a treatment plan and the assessment of treatment effectiveness.

Issues in detecting and monitoring adherence

A number of factors contribute to the difficulty in measuring adherence to medication regimens. One of the major factors is that many times nonadherence is not freely disclosed in clinical practice. This is a crucial problem because the assessment of adherence has largely relied on self-report. Patients infrequently volunteer such information, and when asked, answers may be subject to self-presentational bias. In general, patients tend to want to please their clinician and say what the clinician supposedly wants to hear, which is, "I am taking the medicines exactly as you prescribed!" For most of our patients with mental illnesses, we know this not to be true. Also, we do not know exactly which patients are likely or not likely to share information with their clinicians about their medication nonadherence. In a study of antidepressant adherence by Burra and colleagues,[3] patients were more likely to report nonadherence if they did not have symptom improvement, had sexual side effects, were female, and had limited education. While it may be naive to think patients who "fit the mold" are the ones who will freely discuss their level of nonadherence to their medications, the identification of certain predictors of self-reported nonadherence may facilitate the overall process of assessing and monitoring medication adherence.

Compounding limited disclosure of nonadherence is the tremendous variability in reasons for medication nonadherence in psychiatry, as patient-, clinician-, and medication-related factors can influence patients' decisions not to take medications as prescribed. These factors and their complex relationships make it difficult to measure medication adherence because we simply do not know if a technique is effectively measuring it.

Finally, the big question is "what is an acceptable level of adherence?" Discriminating patients who are adherent versus nonadherent on the basis of a predetermined definition has not been consistent in research studies in psychiatry. Velligan and colleagues[4] noted that in 161 studies, dosage cutoffs ranged from 50% to 90% and categorical classifications ranged from taking any of the prescribed medication to taking nearly every dose. Undoubtedly, clinicians in practice are faced with the same issue. Is a patient with schizophrenia who takes less than 80% of his or her antipsychotic considered nonadherent? Is a patient who skips one week of his or her antipsychotic regimen nonadherent? The lack of a standardized definition poses a problem during the detection and monitoring of medication adherence because there is no explicit standard to which to compare the patient's behavior.

Currently, *there is no "gold standard" technique of measuring adherence,[1] and no one measurement technique is appropriate for each and every clinical setting.* Regardless of which measurement technique is used, it is important to consider its reliability and validity (Table 4.1). With regard to reliability, how consistent is the technique in measuring adherence? With regard to validity, how well does the technique measure adherence? Several types of reliability and validity exist and need to be shown for sound conclusions to be made about the patient's level of adherence to his or her medication regimen.

The measurement of medication adherence may require more than one measurement technique. The use of two or more measurement techniques may

Table 4.1 Validity and Reliability	
Type	**Refers to...**
Validity	
Face validity	Acceptability to respondent
Content validity	Comprehensiveness
Construct validity	Appropriateness for assessing construct
Criterion-related validity	Predictability of future event
Reliability	
Internal consistency	Relationships of individual items with one another
Test–retest reliability	Consistency across time
Intersetting reliability	Consistency across settings
Interrater reliability	Consistency across assessors

address limitations of the respective techniques if used alone and provide corroborative information. It has been suggested that at least one of the measurement techniques should be a direct or objective method (i.e., analysis of biologic fluids, use of a tracer compound, pill counts, prescription records, electronic medication monitoring).[4] For example, a clinician may choose to use self-report and random blood levels to monitor adherence to lithium treatment in a patient with bipolar disorder. While it may be beneficial to capture more data, it is equally important to make sure that the results of each specific technique support one conclusion regarding the patient's extent of medication adherence.

Methods of measuring adherence

"Our patients' nonadherence is our own fault if we do not assess for it in the very people we treat."

—Penny Shel ton, PharmD, CGP, FASCP

Methods of measuring medication adherence can be categorized into direct and indirect methods (Table 4.2). Each has specific advantages and disadvantages that should be considered in the context of individual patients. No measurement technique absolutely confirms ingestion of a medication, but direct methods are typically considered to be more reliable in measuring adherence compared with indirect methods.[5]

Direct methods of measuring adherence

Direct patient observation

Direct patient observation is perhaps the most accurate method of measuring medication adherence. Outside of psychiatry, this method has been largely used in patients with infectious diseases because adherence to treatment regimens is

TAble 4.2 Direct and Indirect Methods of Measuring Adherence

Method	Advantages	Disadvantages
Direct Methods		
Direct patient observation	• Accurate • Noninvasive	• Does not confirm medication ingestion • Impractical
Measurement of drug in blood or urine	• Objective • Quantifiable data	• Affected by patient-specific pharmacokinetics • Expensive • Invasive • Not available for many medications • Only confirms recent medication use
Measurement of biologic marker	• Confirms extended use • Objective • Quantifiable data	• Affected by patient-specific pharmacokinetics • Expensive • Invasive • Susceptible to other factors

TAble 4.2 (Contd.)

Method	Advantages	Disadvantages
Indirect Methods		
Patient self-reports	• Common • Inexpensive • Noninvasive • Quick • Simple	• Inappropriate tone of communication can be problematic • Inconsistent and error-prone over time • Susceptible to self-presentational bias and poor recall
Patient diaries	• Address poor recall • Inexpensive • Medication regimen data • Noninvasive • Quick • Simple	• Diaries need to be returned • Susceptible to self-presentational bias
Adherence questionnaires/ rating scales	• Easy to administer • Noninvasive • Quick • Psychometrically validated	• May require trained interviewer • Susceptible to self-presentational bias and poor recall
Pill counts	• Easy to perform • Inexpensive • Noninvasive • Objective • Quantifiable data	• Patient manipulation of unused medication
Prescription refill records	• Easy to obtain • Long-term data • Noninvasive • Objective	• Does not confirm medication ingestion • May be limited to specific locations • May require database knowledge
Electronic medication monitors	• Provides information on dosing patterns • Noninvasive • Objective • Precise • Quantifiable data	• Does not confirm medication ingestion • Expensive • Inconvenient

a strong predictor of outcomes. The World Health Organization has maintained that directly observed therapy, short course (DOTS) is effective in controlling the spread of tuberculosis (TB).[6] The success of direct observation in increasing treatment adherence and curbing the spread of TB has led to its expansion for other infectious disease states, namely individuals with HIV.[7]

In inpatient psychiatric facilities, direct patient observation may have utility. Having a psychiatric nurse or mental health worker witness a patient swallowing his or her medications may facilitate adherence to psychotropic medications. However, personnel issues may limit an institution's ability for direct patient observation. Furthermore, this method is not infallible, as a patient may "cheek" his or her medication and remove it when free from direct observation.

The feasibility of direct patient observation by health-care practitioners across outpatient clinical settings is relatively limited due to impracticality. While direct patient observation is effective for short-course therapies, such therapies are very uncommon in patients with mental illnesses. However, such supervision by a clinician, nurse, or social worker may not be necessary: relatives of patients with mental illnesses may be a viable option to directly observe psychotropic medication administration. In fact, this relative-based monitoring approach has been shown to improve treatment adherence and reduce disability in individuals with schizophrenia in developing countries.[8]

Measurement of drug in urine or blood

The presence of drug concentrations in urine or blood of patients can serve as a proxy for medication adherence. Concentrations of several psychotropic medications, such as lithium, valproate, tricyclic antidepressants, and clozapine, are routinely determined in clinical practice as part of a therapeutic dosing and monitoring plan. Therapeutic monitoring itself may indirectly improve medication adherence because the patient knows that the clinician will be checking his or her urine or blood.

Drug concentration data have been studied to evaluate a patient's level of adherence. In patients with bipolar disorder, identification of subtherapeutic serum concentrations of lithium, carbamazepine, or valproate may suggest poor adherence. Drotar and colleagues[9] measured adherence to lithium/divalproex combination therapy by the presence or absence of minimum serum concentrations of lithium (0.6 mmol/L) or divalproex (50 mcg/mL) in 107 youths with bipolar disorder. Sixty-six percent of the lithium serum concentrations were in the therapeutic range across the study period, while 84% of the divalproex concentrations were therapeutic.

Monitoring concentrations of antidepressants has also been evaluated as a proxy of adherence in patients with depression. In a 26-month study of 17 depressed patients treated with tricyclic antidepressants, the large variability in plasma concentrations of these agents was partially attributed to nonadherence.[10] Altmura and Mauri[11] found that depressed patients who were informed about their medications had less fluctuation in their tricyclic antidepressant level-dose ratio over a 6-month period compared to those who were not informed, which may have reflected improved adherence. Plasma and saliva drug concentration monitoring of selective serotonin reuptake inhibitors has also been used as a measurement of adherence.[12,13]

Given the high rates of nonadherence with antipsychotic medications seen in patients with schizophrenia, monitoring of antipsychotic concentrations in biologic fluids may be beneficial. Studies evaluating outcomes in patients with schizophrenia have used antipsychotic plasma or urine levels to assess medication adherence.[14,15] Rettenbacher and colleagues[15] used plasma analysis of antipsychotic concentrations in a study of 61 patients with schizophrenia and found 53% to be fully adherent. Unlike with lithium and tricyclic antidepressants, the value of antipsychotic concentrations in biologic fluids as measures for adherence in patients with schizophrenia has not been systematically established. Velligan and colleagues[2] found that plasma concentrations of antipsychotics in outpatients with schizophrenia may not be an optimal method, as plasma levels did not correlate well with other measures of adherence, including pill count and electronic monitoring. Furthermore, most laboratories do not perform such assays.

There are significant limitations in using drug levels in biologic fluids as measures of medication adherence. First, adequate drug levels in biologic fluids do not necessarily mean the patient has been adherent for an extended period of time; it simply indicates that the patient has taken the medication recently. Serial, random measurements of drug concentrations are more likely to provide a better picture of the patient's level of adherence. Second, drug concentrations do not provide information about the timing of doses consumed. Although urine or blood levels of a drug may be considered therapeutic, patients may be erratic in the manner in which they take their medications, suggesting some degree of nonadherence. Third, drug concentrations may be significantly affected by interindividual differences in pharmacokinetics, diet, and co-administration of other medications. Lithium 300 mg twice daily may result in a serum level of 0.8 mEq/L in one patient but 1.2 mEq/L in another. Finally, measurement of drug levels in urine or blood is expensive and invasive and not available for all psychotropic medications. In addition, data about appropriate or therapeutic concentration ranges, which may be used to define adherence, are limited to a handful of psychotropic medications. Despite these limitations, measurement of drug concentrations in biologic fluids may have utility in patients who are suspected to be nonadherent.

Measurement of biologic markers

Adherence may be measured through the use of biologic markers and tracer compounds. Biologic markers may be useful to evaluate adherence over an extended period of time, although they are not a direct measurement of adherence and are expensive and invasive. For example, a number of studies have shown that an elevated HbA1C value in a patient with diabetes mellitus suggests poor glycemic control, which may be attributed to medication nonadherence.[16] In psychiatry, prolactin levels and saccadic eye movements have been shown to be consistent biomarkers of antipsychotic treatment[17]; flicker discrimination, electroencephalography (alpha and beta bands), and rapid eye movement (REM) sleep duration for antidepressant treatment[18]; and saccadic peak velocity and visual analogue scores of alertness for benzodiazepine treatment.[19] However, the usefulness of these markers with regard to the assessment of psychotropic medication adherence has not been determined.

Tracer compounds, such as phenobarbital and digoxin, can be added to a drug and measured in biologic fluids.[1] Like drug concentrations, however, tracer compounds do not provide useful data regarding adherence, are subject to limitations of pharmacokinetic variability, and are expensive and invasive. Kapur and colleagues[20] used riboflavin and urine analysis to assess medication-taking behaviors of patients with schizophrenia and found a high error rate in medication adherence.

Indirect methods of measuring adherence

Patient self-reports and diaries

Self-report measures, which include patient interviews and diaries, are the most common method to measure medication adherence in clinical practice. In research, self-report of medication adherence has been the most widely used method. In a review of studies assessing adherence to oral antipsychotics, Velligan and colleagues[4] reported that self-report was used alone or in combination with another measurement technique in 66% of the studies. Self-report has also been used to assess medication adherence across other psychiatric disorders, including depression.[3] There has been considerable variability in the specifics of the self-report methods (e.g., unstructured versus structured interviews, patient diaries, medication checklists) across studies.[4] The concordance of a self-report method with a direct or objective measure of adherence varies, with patient questionnaires and diaries having a higher degree of concordance than patient interviews.[4]

While these techniques are simple, inexpensive, and practical in the clinical setting, they are not very reliable ways to accurately measure adherence because of several potential confounds. First, patients may misrepresent their true level of adherence in order to please their clinicians, and this usually results in an over-estimation. Second, memory recall may be an issue with self-reporting. This may be especially true in patients with a psychiatric illness, as cognitive deficits are associated with many disorders. Assessing recent (i.e., past 24 to 48 hours) adherence through self-reporting techniques may have better reliability and validity compared with more distant (i.e., 1 to 2 months) assessments. Third, the relationship between the interviewer and patient and the manner of communication may have a significant impact on self-report measures. Negative wording of questions about medication adherence may be interpreted as blame by the patient. It is important to frame the interview questions in a nonthreatening manner. Finally, patient interviews are often conducted without a structured set of questions, making this self-report technique vulnerable to inconsistency from visit to visit.

"PLEASE tell me that you took your medications as I prescribed" versus

"Do you have any medications for which you sometimes miss taking a dose?"

Adherence questionnaires and rating scales

General adherence questionnaires and rating scales have been developed to address some of the limitations associated with self-reporting techniques. These measures are psychometrically tested and have shown good reliability and validity. For example, Svarstad and colleagues[21] developed the Brief Medication Questionnaire (BMQ), a self-report tool for screening adherence and barriers to adherence. The BMQ consists of a five-item Regimen Screen that assesses how patients took each medication in the past week; a two-item Belief Screen that assesses drug effects and bothersome features; and a two-item Recall Screen that assesses memory recall. The BMQ was found to be sensitive for repeat and sporadic medication nonadherence.[21]

Another example of a general adherence questionnaire is the Medication Adherence Questionnaire (MAQ) developed by Morisky and colleagues.[22] Although the MAQ's accuracy in predicting poor adherence is low, it has been validated for use in patients with psychiatric disorders.[23]

Adherence rating scales have also been developed for specific psychiatric conditions, namely schizophrenia. The Medication Adherence Rating Scale (MARS)[24] was originally developed to evaluate adherence in patients with psychoses, but it has been successfully used in patients with bipolar disorder.[25] The Drug Attitude Inventory (DAI)[26] and the Rating of Medication Influences (ROMI)[27] have been psychometrically tested and are frequently used to assess reasons for adherence and nonadherence to medications in patients with schizophrenia.

More recently, the Brief Adherence Rating Scale (BARS) was developed to measure adherence to oral antipsychotic medications. The BARS is a brief, pencil-and-paper, clinician-administered adherence instrument consisting of four items: number of prescribed doses per day (question 1); number of days, over the past month, the patient did not take the prescribed doses (question 2); number of days, over the past month, the patient took less than the prescribed doses (question 3); and an overall visual analogue rating scale to assess the proportion of doses taken by the patient in the past month (0% to 100%).[28] In a recent study of its psychometric properties in 61 outpatients with schizophrenia or schizoaffective disorder, the BARS showed a positive correlation with electronic medication monitoring, as well as high internal and test–retest reliability.[28] The BARS showed good concurrent validity with the Positive and Negative Syndrome Scale (PANSS) (i.e., the higher the mean BARS adherence score, the lower the mean PANSS total and positive subscale scores), and its sensitivity and specificity were acceptable in terms of identifying nonadherent patients. The brevity and ease of administration of the BARS suggests feasibility and usefulness in the community setting.[28]

Pill counts

The simplicity and low cost of pill counting make it an attractive method to measure medication adherence, and indeed pill counting is commonly used in clinical practice and research settings. Rosenheck and colleagues[29] evaluated medication continuation and compliance in patients with schizophrenia receiving clozapine or haloperidol using pill counting. Although patients on clozapine had a significantly longer duration of medication continuation compared to those on haloperidol, there was no difference between groups in medication compliance.[29]

Pill counting, however, is not considered a reliable method to assess adherence as it typically tends to overestimate. Medications may be switched between bottles, or even "dumped," to make it seem as if adherence is high. Furthermore, pill counting does not provide information about patterns of nonadherence, such as timing of missed doses or reasons for nonadherence.

Prescription refill records

With the advent of computerized pharmacy databases, the use of prescription refill records to assess medication adherence has increased. This method evaluates the assumed use of medications based on refill patterns in a closed pharmacy system (Table 4.3). A number of measures of medication adherence can be calculated from pharmacy records or databases, including compliance rate (CR); continuous measure of medication acquistion (CMA); continuous measure of medication gaps (CMG); continuous, multiple-interval measure of oversupply (CMOS); continuous, single-interval measure of medication availability (CSA); days between fills adherence rate (DBR); medication possession ratio (MPR); medication possession ratio, modified (MPRm); medication refill adherence (MRA); proportion of days covered (PDC); and refill compliance rate (RCR).[30] These calculations are applicable to any psychiatric disorder.

Of course, patients may refill a prescription outside the system, which affects the accuracy of adherence estimates. In addition, this method requires that the database be complete and accurate with regard to prescribing and dispensing information. Despite these limitations, pharmacy refill records and databases have been frequently used to assess medication adherence across various psychiatric disorders. Dolder and colleagues[31] used CMG and the compliant fill rate (the number of prescription fills indicating adherence in relation to the total number of prescription fills) at 6 and 12 months to compare adherence in patients with schizophrenia receiving atypical versus typical antipsychotics. Six- and 12-month adherence rates were higher in patients receiving atypical antipsychotics. CMG ratios were 14% for atypical antipsychotics and 23% for typical antipsychotics at 12 months; compliant fill rates were 55% for atypical antipsychotics and 50% for typical antipsychotics at 12 months.[31] Gilmer and colleagues[32] used cumulative MPR to evaluate antipsychotic adherence, service utilization, and treatment costs in Medicaid enrollees with schizophrenia. Underuse and overuse of antipsychotic medications were noted, as 40% were found to be nonadherent or partially adherent and 19% were excess fillers. Patients who were found to be adherent had lower rates of psychiatric hospitalization and associated hospitalization costs than nonadherent patients.

Table 4.3 Measures Used to Assess Medication Adherence from Pharmacy Records[30]

Measure	Meaning of Value	Calculation	Comments
CMA	Adherence for cumulative time period	Days' supply obtained throughout observation period/number of days of observation	
CMG	Nonadherence for cumulative time period	Total days of treatment gaps*/number of days of observation	0 = complete adherence, 1 = complete nonadherence
CMOS	Nonadherence for cumulative time period	Total days of treatment gaps (or surplus)/total days in observation	Allows for surplus
CR	Adherence for period between dispensations	(Days' supplies minus days' supply of last dispensation)/number of days from first dispensation up to last dispensation × 100	Does not require end date of observation
CSA	Adherence for observation period	Days' supply of dispensation/number of days from dispensation up to next dispensation	
DBR	Overall adherence percentage	1—([Number of days between dispensations—total days' supply]/number of days between dispensations) × 100	
MPR	Ratio of medication available	Total days' supply : number of days of observation	
MPRm	Adherence percentage	Total days' supply/(number of days from first dispensation up to last dispensation + days' supply of last dispensation) × 100	Includes final dispensation period
MRA	Overall adherence percentage	Total days' supply/number of days of observation × 100	
PDC	Percentage of days with medication available	Total days' supply/number of days of observation × 100	Capped at 100%
RCR	Overall adherence percentage	(Total days' supply × 100)/number of days from first to last dispensation	

*Treatment gaps = Total days of observation—total days' supply.[36-38]

Adherence studies in depression and ADHD have also used MPR to show poor rates of adherence with treatment regimens and corresponding outcomes.[33,34]

Electronic medication monitors

Electronic medication monitors (EMMs) are normal pill bottles with a special cap with a microchip that registers the date and time of every bottle opening (Fig. 4.1). Blister-pack EMMs have also been recently developed. EMM technology provides a more accurate, detailed assessment of medication adherence. Information from EMMs is typically downloaded during a return visit and analyzed for patterns of presumed medication use. Although EMMs do not provide information directly on medication ingestion (i.e., if and how), they can supplement data from other methods of adherence measurement.[35] Early EMMs were expensive, prone to malfunction, and burdensome to use, limiting their use in routine clinical practice. However, recent advances in printed electronics and manufacturing scaled to larger multi-year clinical studies using blister EMMs, as well as integration of EMMs into off-the-shelf pharmacy vials, such as Rexam's 1-Clic®, are rapidly paving the way to wider adoption. It should be noted that patients may initially show reactivity bias when EMMs are used.

Medication Event Monitoring System (MEMS®), the eCAP, and Med-ic® ECM© are among the EMMs available for use. The MEMS® consists of a standard pill bottle cap that has a computer chip within. The computer chip records the time at which the bottle is opened by the patient to remove the tablet or capsule, thereby providing reliable data on individual dosing patterns. The Rexam is similar to the MEMS cap and tracks medication usage through a microprocessor embedded into a Rexam 1-Clic® bottle cap. The Med-ic® ECM© (Electronic Compliance Monitor) is a device that provides inventory control for blister-packaged medications. The Med-ic® ECM© records the time each pill or capsule is expelled from the blister package, keeping a log of medication use.

Electronic monitoring in psychiatry

The majority of research studies in psychiatry have used self-reporting or clinician reporting as the method of measuring adherence to medications. Specifically in schizophrenia, subjective and indirect methods (i.e., self-report, provider report, significant other report, and chart review) have been used in more than 75% of studies.[4] In search of a more reliable method to assess medication adherence in patients with psychiatric disorders, researchers have been examining the utility of electronic medication monitoring. Studies have examined MEMS® caps as a method of measuring medication adherence in patients with schizophrenia or schizoaffective disorder,[36] depression,[37] and substance dependence.[38] Overall, MEMS® caps have been shown to be a reliable method of assessing adherence compared with other indirect and direct measures (Table 4.4).

Selecting a method of measuring adherence for your patient

An ideal measurement tool for medication adherence would allow accurate determination of a patient's level of medication adherence and would have optimal feasibility across all clinical settings (Table 4.5).[39]

Unfortunately, there is no foolproof method that will guarantee the detection of medication adherence or nonadherence in patients. Clinicians should

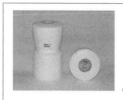

Figure 4.1 Electronic medication monitors. (Left) The MEMS® cap from AARDEX, © 2008, AARDEX Ltd. Reproduced with permission. (Middle) eCAP from IMC, Copyright 2008, Information Mediary Corporation (IMC). Reproduced with permission. (Right) Med-ic® ECM© from IMC. Copyright 2008, Information Mediary Corporation (IMC). Reproduced with permission.

Table 4.4 Key Studies of Electronic Medication Monitors in Psychiatry[36–38]

Reference	Methods	Results
36	Antipsychotics for schizophrenia or schizoaffective disorder (n = 61) MEMS® vs. self-report vs. clinician report vs. research assistant report	MEMS® detected greater rates of nonadherence (57%) than self-report (5%) or clinician report (7%) MEMS® comparable to research assistant report (54%), though some disagreement (36%)
37	MEMS® to estimate 6-month adherence to antidepressants in major depressive disorder (n = 85)	70% had overall adherence above 80% Lower adherence in dropouts (70%) versus completers (84%)
38	Naltrexone for alcohol dependence (n = 93) MEMS® vs. pill count	Pill count (88%) yielded higher estimate of adherence than MEMS® (80%) MEMS® more consistently correlated with treatment outcomes

Table 4.5 Ideal Characteristics of an Adherence Measurement Method[39]

• Provides quantitative data over a period of time (not simply "adherent" or "nonadherent")
• Inexpensive
• Reliable
• Objective
• Easy to use

weigh the characteristics of each available method, both positive and negative, in relation to what they are trying to achieve and what resources are available. For example, if a clinician wants to determine whether a patient with schizophrenia is taking his or her antipsychotic medication twice daily as instructed, the use of a MEMS® cap or o ther electronic monitoring device that provides timing data would be appropriate. Clinicians should strive to use more than one strategy to monitor medication adherence, and should implement such strategies early in the treatment process.

References

1. Osterberg L, Blaschke T. Adherence to medication. *N Engl J Med*. 2005;353: 487–497.

2. Velligan DI, Wang M, Diamond P, et al. Relationships among subjective and objective measures of adherence to oral antipsychotic medications. *Psychiatr Serv*. 2007;58:1187–1192.

3. Burra TA, Chen E, McIntyre RS, Grace SL, Blackmore ER, Stewart DE. Predictors of self-reported antidepressant adherence. *Behav Med*. 2007;32:127–134.

4. Velligan DI, Lam YW, Glahn DC, et al. Defining and assessing adherence to oral antipsychotics: a review of the literature. Schizophr Bull. 2006;32:724–742.

5. Bond WS, Hussar DA. Detection methods and strategies for improving medication compliance. *Am J Hosp Pharm*. 1991;48:1978–1988.

6. Burman WJ, Dalton CB, Cohn DL, Butler JR, Reves RR. A cost-effectiveness analysis of directly observed therapy vs. self-administered therapy for treatment of tuberculosis. Chest. 1997;112:63–70.

7. Mitty JA, Macalino G, Taylor L, Harwell JI, Flanigan TP. Directly observed therapy (DOT) for individuals with HIV: successes and challenges. *MedGenMed*. 2003;5:30.

8. Chatterjee S, Patel V, Chatterjee A, Weiss HA. Evaluation of a community-based rehabilitation model for chronic schizophrenia in rural India. *Br J Psychiatry*. 2003;182:57–62.

9. Drotar D, Greenley RN, Demeter CA, et al. Adherence to pharmacological treatment for juvenile bipolar disorder. *J Am Acad Child Adolesc Psychiatry*. 2007;46:831–839.

10. Loo H, Benyacoub AK, Rovei V, Altamura CA, Vadrot M, Morselli PL. Long-term monitoring of tricyclic antidepressant plasma concentrations. *Br J Psychiatry*. 1980;137:444–451.

11. Altamura AC, Mauri M. Plasma concentrations, information and therapy adherence during long-term treatment with antidepressants. *Br J Clin Pharmacol*. 1985;20:714–716.

12. Akerblad AC, Bengtsson F, Ekselius L, von Knorring L. Effects of an educational compliance enhancement programme and therapeutic drug monitoring on treatment adherence in depressed patients managed by general practitioners. *Int Clin Psychopharmacol*. 2003;18:347–354.

13. Tsuruta T, Yang C, Ueki H, et al. Determination of paroxetine in human saliva by reversed-phase high-performance liquid chromatography with UV detection. Nihon Shinkei Seishin Yakurigaku Zasshi. 2007;27:9–12.

14. Falloon IR, Boyd JL, McGill CW, et al. Family management in the prevention of morbidity of schizophrenia. Clinical outcome of a two-year longitudinal study. *Arch Gen Psychiatry*. 1985;42:887–896.

15. Rettenbacher MA, Hofer A, Eder U, et al. Compliance in schizophrenia: psychopathology, side effects, and patients' attitudes toward the illness and medication. *J Clin Psychiatry*. 2004;65:1211–1218.

16. Krapek K, King K, Warren SS, et al. Medication adherence and associated hemoglobin A1c in type 2 diabetes. Ann Pharmacother. 2004;38:1357–1362.

17. de Visser SJ, van der Post J, Pieters MS, Cohen AF, van Gerven JM. Biomarkers for the effects of antipsychotic drugs in healthy volunteers. *Br J Clin Pharmacol.* 2001;51:119–132.

18. Dumont GJ, de Visser SJ, Cohen AF, van Gerven JM. Biomarkers for the effects of selective serotonin reuptake inhibitors (SSRIs) in healthy subjects. *Br J Clin Pharmacol.* 2005;59:495–510.

19. de Visser SJ, van der Post JP, de Waal PP, Cornet F, Cohen AF, van Gerven JM. Biomarkers for the effects of benzodiazepines in healthy volunteers. *Br J Clin Pharmacol.* 2003;55:39–50.

20. Kapur S, Ganguli R, Ulrich R, Raghu U. Use of random-sequence riboflavin as a marker of medication compliance in chronic schizophrenics. *Schizophr Res.* 1991;6:49–53.

21. Svarstad BL, Chewning BA, Sleath BL, Claesson C. The Brief Medication Questionnaire: a tool for screening patient adherence and barriers to adherence. *Patient Educ Couns.* 1999;37:113–124.

22. Morisky DE, Green LW, Levine DM. Concurrent and predictive validity of a self-reported measure of medication adherence. *Med Care.* 1986;24:67–74.

23. Fialko L, Garety PA, Kuipers E, et al. A large-scale validation study of the Medication Adherence Rating Scale (MARS). *Schizophr Res.* 2008;100:53–59.

24. hompson K, Kulkarni J, Sergejew AA. Reliability and validity of a new Medication Adherence Rating Scale (MARS) for the psychoses. *Schizophr Res.* 2000;42:241–247.

25. Rosa AR, Marco M, Fachel JM, Kapczinski F, Stein AT, Barros HM. Correlation between drug treatment adherence and lithium treatment attitudes and knowledge by bipolar patients. Prog Neuropsychopharmacol Biol Psychiatry. 2007;31:217–224.

26. Hogan TP, Awad AG, Eastwood R. A self-report scale predictive of drug compliance in schizophrenics: reliability and discriminative validity. *Psychol Med.* 1983;13:177–183.

27. Weiden P, Rapkin B, Mott T, et al. Rating of Medication Influences (ROMI) scale in schizophrenia. *Schizophr Bull.* 1994;20:297–310.

28. Byerly MJ, Nakonezny PA, Rush AJ. The Brief Adherence Rating Scale (BARS) validated against electronic monitoring in assessing the antipsychotic medication adherence of outpatients with schizophrenia and schizoaffective disorder. *Schizophr Res.* 2008;100:60–69.

29. Rosenheck R, Chang S, Choe Y, et al. Medication continuation and compliance: a comparison of patients treated with clozapine and haloperidol. *J Clin Psychiatry.* 2000;61:382–386.

30. Hess LM, Raebel MA, Conner DA, Malone DC. Measurement of adherence in pharmacy administrative databases: a proposal for standard definitions and preferred measures. *Ann Pharmacother.* 2006;40:1280–1288.

31. Dolder CR, Lacro JP, Dunn LB, Jeste DV. Antipsychotic medication adherence: is there a difference between typical and atypical agents? *Am J Psychiatry.* 2002;159:103–108.

32. Gilmer TP, Dolder CR, Lacro JP, et al. Adherence to treatment with antipsychotic medication and health care costs among Medicaid beneficiaries with schizophrenia. *Am J Psychiatry.* 2004;161:692–699.

33. Akincigil A, Bowblis JR, Levin C, Walkup JT, Jan S, Crystal S. Adherence to antidepressant treatment among privately insured patients diagnosed with depression. *Med Care.* 2007;45:363–369.

34. Perwien A, Hall J, Swensen A, Swindle R. Stimulant treatment patterns and compliance in children and adults with newly treated attention-deficit/hyperactivity disorder. *J Manag Care Pharm.* 2004;10:122–129.

35. Cramer JA. Microelectronic systems for monitoring and enhancing patient compliance with medication regimens. Drugs. 1995;49:321–327.

36. Byerly MJ, Thompson A, Carmody T, et al. Validity of electronically monitored medication adherence and conventional adherence measures in schizophrenia. *Psychiatr Serv.* 2007;58:844–847.

37. Demyttenaere K, Adelin A, Patrick M, Walthere D, Katrien de B, Michele S. Six-month compliance with antidepressant medication in the treatment of major depressive disorder. *Int Clin Psychopharmacol.* 2008;23:36–42.

38. Namkoong K, Farren CK, O'Connor PG, O'Malley SS. Measurement of compliance with naltrexone in the treatment of alcohol dependence: research and clinical implications. *J Clin Psychiatry.* 1999;60:449–453.

39. Farmer KC. Methods for measuring and monitoring medication regimen adherence in clinical trials and clinical practice. *Clin Ther.* 1999;21:1074–1090.

Chapter 5

Pharmacological options for managing nonadherence

Optimal treatment outcomes are rarely achieved when a "one-size-fits-all" approach is used. The success of pharmacological treatment for any illness relies on a multitude of factors, including drug administration, efficacy, safety, and tolerability. Such issues with pharmacological treatment regimens may have a profound effect on medication adherence. Thus, careful management of medication-related issues, many of which may lead to partial or full medication nonadherence, is imperative to minimize the likelihood of suboptimal treatment outcomes. One manner in which to address medication-related issues is through various pharmacological options.

Pharmacological options for the management of medication adherence have evolved considerably through innovations in the drug development process. Novel agents have been developed to address limitations of existing medications, namely with regard to side effect profiles. Novel drug dosage forms and delivery systems have also been developed to enhance medication adherence. Advantages of novel formulations with regard to promotion of adherence include ease of administration, minimized fluctuations in drug concentrations, reduced dosing frequency, reduced risk of side effects, and simplification of dosing regimens (Table 5.1).

Table 5.1 Advantages/Disadvantages of Drug Delivery Systems in Terms of Adherence

Drug Delivery System	Advantages	Disadvantages
Extended-, sustained-release tablets/capsules	• Minimized drug concentration fluctuations • Reduced dosing frequency • Reduced side effect burden	• Cannot crush, chew, or divide some tablets/capsules
Orally disintegrating tablets	• Easier to swallow • Immediate administration (no need for water)	• Difficult to handle without breaking into small pieces • More costly than conventional oral tablets • Unpleasant taste
Chewable tablets	• Easier to swallow • May be preferred for children	• Unpleasant taste

Table 5.1 *(Contd.)*		
Drug Delivery System	**Advantages**	**Disadvantages**
Fixed-dose combination tablets/capsules	• Simplified regimen	• Difficult to adjust dose of one medication
Oral solutions	• Easier to swallow • Immediate administration (no need for water)	• Dosing inaccuracies • Inconvenient to store • Physical instability • Unpleasant texture
Transdermal patches	• Minimized drug concentration fluctuations • Reduced dosing frequency • Reduced side effect burden • Used if difficulty in swallowing	• Inadvertently may fall off • Skin irritation • Some cannot be immersed in water • Some may be visible
Long-acting injections	• Minimized drug concentration fluctuations • Reduced dosing frequency • Reduced side effect burden	• Inability to rapidly discontinue medication if necessary • Injection pain • Stigma
Implants	• Minimized drug concentration fluctuations • Reduced dosing frequency • Reduced side effect burden	• Informed consent may be required • Surgical procedure to place or remove

Improved adherence through novel drug delivery in medicine

New drug dosage forms and delivery systems have had a significant impact on medication adherence across medicine. In some disease states, such as HIV/acquired immunodeficiency syndrome (AIDS), hypertension, and diabetes, there is convincing evidence that increased dosing frequency and complexity of medication regimen are associated with poor rates of adherence. Medication formulations that have reduced the number and frequency of pills taken daily and have improved ease of administration have been shown to improve overall adherence rates to pharmacotherapy in patients with various chronic medical conditions. In addition, formulations that reduce the dosing frequency have also been associated with a more favorable side effect profile. For example, twice-daily dosing of HAART has been associated with higher rates of adherence than thrice-daily dosing in patients with HIV/AIDS.[1] In a meta-analysis of dose frequency and adherence to antihypertensives in over 11,000 subjects, Iskedjian and colleagues[2] reported improved adherence rates with once-daily dosing. Specifically, the mean adherence rate for once-daily dosing (91%) was significantly higher than for twice-daily (87%) or multiple-daily (83%) dosing. Administration of combination products, such as metformin/rosiglitazone and metformin/glyburide, has been associated with higher adherence rates (77%) compared with administration of the agents separately (54%).[3]

Improving adherence through novel drug delivery in psychiatry

As our understanding of the overall management of psychiatric disorders has grown, psychotropic medications with novel mechanisms of action or formulations have been introduced to the market. While there have not necessarily been significant advances in terms of treatment efficacy, newer psychotropic agents generally are considered to have a more favorable side effect profile than their older counterparts. New formulations of psychotropic medications have also been developed to improve tolerability and address issues related to medication nonadherence. *The decision of which psychotropic medication to use should be that of both the clinician and patient and should depend on the patient's past experiences with specific medications, the patient's preference of medications, and a thorough evaluation of benefit–risk profiles.*

Antipsychotics

Improving medication adherence through innovation in drug development in schizophrenia has rightfully been devoted a great deal of attention. Rational use of atypical antipsychotics may confer benefit with regard to medication adherence. Furthermore, use of long-acting injectable antipsychotic formulations, as well as controlled-release, liquid oral, and rapidly dissolving tablet formulations, may improve medication adherence.

Typical versus atypical antipsychotics

Both typical and atypical antipsychotics are effective in reducing positive symptoms, while atypical antipsychotics may be more effective in treating negative symptoms. Atypical antipsychotics show an improved side effect profile compared to typical antipsychotics, particularly with regard to extrapyramidal symptoms and tardive dyskinesia. However, atypical antipsychotics tend to cause significant weight gain and other metabolic disturbances.

It has been suggested that adherence to atypical antipsychotics may be better than that to typical antipsychotics due to improved patient tolerability. Dolder and colleagues[4] evaluated adherence to antipsychotic regimens using pharmacy refill records in patients receiving haloperidol, perphenazine, risperidone, olanzapine, and quetiapine. They found moderately higher rates of adherence at 6 and 12 months in patients receiving atypical antipsychotics compared to those receiving typical antipsychotics (6 months: 57% vs. 50%; 12 months: 55% vs. 50%).[4] Among veterans with schizophrenia or schizoaffective disorder, Valenstein and colleagues[5] reported higher rates of poor adherence, defined as a medication possession ratio less than 0.8, in patients receiving atypical antipsychotics (42%) than those receiving typical antipsychotics (38%). Clearly, there is no consensus whether one antipsychotic class is better when it comes to adherence, and the discontinuation findings from CATIE[6] support this.

As observed in CATIE, lack of efficacy and poor tolerability were among the most common reasons for antipsychotic discontinuation.[6] If therapy with one particular antipsychotic is ineffective or intolerable, switching to another agent may provide improved symptom control and tolerability. This may, in turn, improve adherence to the antipsychotic treatment. The choice of which antipsychotic to switch to will depend on the reasons for nonadherence with the original antipsychotic, as well as patient characteristics and preferences (Table 5.2).

Antipsychotic doses and dosing frequency have been shown to be predictors of adherence.[7] Excessive antipsychotic dose is likely to result in increased risk

Table 5.2 Examples of Optimizing Antipsychotic Therapy Through Switching

Reason for Nonadherence	Switch to...
Lack of efficacy	
Continued positive symptoms	Another atypical or typical antipsychotic
Continued negative symptoms	Another atypical antipsychotic
Poor tolerability	
Anticholinergic side effects	Aripiprazole, haloperidol, paliperidone, quetiapine, risperidone, ziprasidone
Extrapyramidal symptoms	Clozapine, quetiapine
Sexual side effects	Aripiprazole, clozapine, quetiapine, ziprasidone
Weight gain/metabolic effects	Aripiprazole, haloperidol, paliperidone, perphenazine, quetiapine, risperidone, ziprasidone

of adverse effects; thus, simply reducing the antipsychotic dose may improve tolerability and adherence. It is important to maintain a minimally effective dose to provide adequate symptom control. Antipsychotics that can be administered once daily may also improve adherence. Most antipsychotics have long half-lives of 20 hours or more, which allows for once-daily dosing. Quetiapine and ziprasidone have shorter half-lives, thus possibly requiring multiple dosing during the course of the day. Chengappa and colleagues[8] examined the feasibility of switching patients with schizophrenia or schizoaffective disorder who are stable on twice-daily dosing of quetiapine to once-daily dosing, and found the switch to be associated with no loss of efficacy. A few patients (15%) experienced symptom worsening and orthostasis when switched to a once-daily quetiapine regimen.[8]

Optimization of antipsychotic treatment through formulations
Adherence may be poor despite efforts to optimize an oral antipsychotic regimen through appropriate drug selection and dosing. In such cases, clinicians should consider the use of alternative formulations of antipsychotics, such as controlled-release, liquid, orally disintegrating, and long-acting injectable preparations. These formulations may offer distinct advantages over traditional oral formulations by addressing relevant determinants of nonadherence.

Controlled-release formulations may improve adherence through convenience (i.e., reduced dosing frequency) and improved tolerability. An extended-release formulation of quetiapine was recently introduced to the market, and once-daily dosing is recommended with this product. Switching to extended-release quetiapine from immediate-release antipsychotics has been shown to be associated with maintained symptom control and improved tolerability.[9] Similarly, paliperidone extended-release uses an osmotic-controlled release oral-delivery system technology to enable once-daily dosing and provide smoother plasma levels for improved tolerability.[10]

Liquid or rapidly dissolving tablet formulations may be beneficial in patients who have difficulty swallowing or who are suspected of "cheeking" their medications. In addition, these preparations may be used in the acute management of agitated patients who refuse intramuscular antipsychotic medication. Oral liquid solutions are available for most typical antipsychotics and for aripiprazole and risperidone. Rapidly dissolving tablets are available for aripiprazole, clozapine, olanzapine, and risperidone. Liquid and rapidly dissolving tablet formulations have generally shown similar bioequivalence and pharmacokinetics to the traditional tablet formulations. In a 6-week, open-label study of olanzapine in 85 patients with schizophrenia or schizoaffective disorder, the rapidly dissolving formulation was found to significantly improve adherence as well as patient attitude and acceptance of medications.[10]

Compared to oral formulations, long-acting injectable (LAI) formulations of fluphenazine, haloperidol, and risperidone are advantageous with respect to medication adherence. First and foremost, LAI antipsychotics improve medication adherence by ensuring the delivery of an antipsychotic medication. With oral antipsychotics, nonadherence can go undetected and then result in a relapse of symptoms. With LAIs, nonadherence is easy to detect, as a patient simply does not come to the clinic for the antipsychotic injection. If a patient does miss an injection, appropriate interventions by the clinical team can be made in a timely fashion to prevent exacerbation of symptomatology. Furthermore, the long half-lives of LAIs ensure that some antipsychotic medication will remain in the patient's body weeks thereafter. Second, improved medication adherence with LAIs may translate into a reduced risk of relapse. In a recent review, Schooler[11] reported a 27% 1-year relapse rate with depot antipsychotics and a 42% rate with oral antipsychotics. Furthermore, use of LAI antipsychotics has been associated with a greater improvement in global functioning compared to oral antipsychotics.[12] Third, LAI antipsychotic formulations avoid first-pass metabolism, which reduces pharmacokinetic variability and results in predictable and stable plasma concentrations. This allows for the lowest effective dose to be used, which reduces the frequency of side effects, including extrapyramidal symptoms.[10] Finally, use of LAIs offers convenience to patients, as they are not required to take antipsychotic medications on a daily basis.

Despite these benefits, LAI antipsychotics are underused in clinical practice settings due to clinician and patient concerns.[13] Clinicians may be reluctant to use LAIs due to the inability to withdraw medication if an adverse effect occurs. While this is true, there is no conclusive evidence indicating that LAI antipsychotics are associated with a greater risk of extrapyramidal symptoms, tardive dyskinesia, or neuroleptic malignant syndrome compared with oral antipsychotics.[10] LAI risperidone may also alleviate such concerns, as the risk of antipsychotic-induced movement disorders is more often attributed to typical antipsychotics.

Patients may prefer not to use LAI formulations because they may feel as if they lose autonomy over their treatment. Patients may also feel labeled as "noncompliant" or "uncooperative" if they are receiving a LAI antipsychotic. Although LAIs are sometimes administered coercively to nonadherent patients, this is not the case for most: the main indication for LAI antipsychotics is maintenance treatment and relapse prevention. A systematic review of survey data from multiple studies showed that a high percentage of patients on LAIs are indeed very satisfied with their current treatment,[14] indicating that experience with LAI antipsychotics may improve a patient's attitude toward this specific formulation (Table 5.3). Another patient concern is discomfort with the injection. LAIs may be associated with pain, redness, and swelling. *Patient acceptance is critical for the successful use of LAI antipsychotics.*

Antidepressants

Poor adherence during the early course of treatment is fairly common in patients receiving antidepressants. Complicated regimens, intolerable side effects, and delayed onset of action are among the most commonly reported reasons for antidepressant discontinuation.[10] New formulations of existing antidepressant medications, including extended-release, rapidly dissolving, and transdermal

Table 5.3 Attitudes Toward Long-Acting Injectable Antipsychotics

Group	Why to Use...	Why Not to Use...
Patients	• Better protection against relapse • Convenient and easier • Improves relationship with clinician • Improved quality of life • Reduced side effects	• Cost • Loss of autonomy • Pain from injection • Stigma
Clinicians	• Easier adherence monitoring • Lower antipsychotic dose • Patient nonadherent to oral formulations • Reduced risk of relapse	• Cost • First-episode patient • High EPS risk with LAI typical antipsychotics • Inability to rapidly discontinue if adverse event occurs • Patient adherent to oral formulations • Patient needs antipsychotic not available as LAI • Patient refusal of LAI • Poorer control of effect than oral formulations

preparations, have been developed to address these issues. As a result, improved adherence may lead to better antidepressant treatment outcomes.

Optimization of antidepressant treatment through formulations

A patient's medication regimen can easily be simplified through the use of controlled-release antidepressant formulations. These products, including controlled-release fluvoxamine, controlled-release paroxetine, extended-release bupropion, extended-release venlafaxine, and once-weekly fluoxetine, allow for convenience. The simplified dosing regimen is believed to improve overall adherence, although a limited number of studies have systematically compared adherence between controlled-release and immediate-release antidepressants. In a 3-month study comparing adherence to daily or weekly fluoxetine in 117 depressed adults, adherence to once-weekly fluoxetine treatment (86%) was higher than that to once-daily fluoxetine (79%). Furthermore, adherence rates declined over time in the daily fluoxetine group, whereas adherence rates remained stable in the weekly fluoxetine group (Fig. 5.1).[10]

Many patients who prematurely discontinue antidepressant treatment do so because of poor tolerability. Controlled-release formulations may be associated with reduced adverse effects compared to immediate-release formulations, because these formulations reduce the peak plasma concentrations seen with immediate-release formulations. Extended-release venlafaxine and controlled-release paroxetine have been shown to have more favorable side effect profiles, particularly with regard to nausea.[10] Similarly, sustained- and extended-release bupropion are associated with a reduced risk of seizures and overall improved tolerability compared with the immediate-release preparation. These formulations of bupropion may be preferred when antidepressant-induced sexual dysfunction,

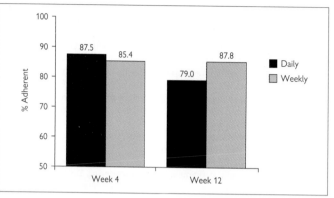

Figure 5.1 Adherence rates of daily versus once-weekly fluoxetine. Information adapted from Claxton A, de Klerk E, Parry M, Robinson JM, Schmidt ME. Patient compliance to a new enteric-coated weekly formulation of fluoxetine during continuation treatment of major depressive disorder. *J Clin Psychiatry* 2000;61:928–932.)

weight gain, and somnolence may be issues negatively affecting adherence.[15] In contrast, no significant improvement in tolerability has been reported with weekly fluoxetine.[10]

An orally disintegrating formulation of mirtazapine (mirtazapine SolTab®) may be useful for patients who have difficulty swallowing. In addition, it has been suggested that this formulation of mirtazapine may be associated with a faster onset of antidepressant activity. This characteristic may be beneficial for those patients who tend to discontinue antidepressant medication due to lack of efficacy early in the treatment course. In an 8-week, randomized, double-blind study of orally disintegrating mirtazapine and sertraline in 345 patients with major depression, mirtazapine was significantly more effective than sertraline at all assessments during the first 2 weeks of the study. Response and remission rates with orally disintegrating mirtazapine were also significantly higher at week 2 compared with sertraline. Thereafter, efficacy was similar in both groups.[10]

Recently, a transdermal delivery system of selegiline has been developed to preferentially inhibit brain monoamine oxidase (MAO) enzymes and avoid the interaction with gastrointestinal MAO enzymes. In doing so, the potential for the well-known drug–food interaction with selegiline and tyramine-containing foods is greatly reduced. Clinical trials of transdermal selegiline in patients with major depression have shown a reduction in the typical side effects associated with MAO inhibitors, which may translate into improved adherence.[10]

Mood stabilizers/anticonvulsants

Part of what makes full adherence in bipolar disorder difficult to achieve is that many patients do not achieve adequate mood stabilization on one medication alone. Because polypharmacy is often necessary, bipolar patients are exposed to complex medication regimens. Thus, medications that are convenient for the patient to take, such as once-a-day dosing formulations, can be very helpful in improving adherence. These formulations also can provide consistent blood levels and reduce the risk of adverse effects.

Divalproex is among the most commonly used mood stabilizers/anticonvulsants in the treatment of patients with bipolar disorder. A delayed-release (DR) formulation of divalproex allows for improved tolerability compared to valproic acid. However, divalproex DR requires twice-daily dosing, which can negatively affect adherence. An extended-release (ER) preparation of divalproex was developed to allow for routine once-daily dosing and improved tolerability due to reduced fluctuations in valproic acid concentrations. In a retrospective chart review, Minirth and Neal[16] reported that a majority of patients (62%) who were switched to divalproex ER from divalproex DR preferred the ER formulation. Sixteen patients (52%) showed clinical improvement after switching to divalproex ER, while 3 (9%) showed clinical deterioration. Switching to divalproex ER was associated with improved tolerability, as 25 (81%) reported either no side effects or no increase in side effects. Six (19%) patients reported one new side effect, particularly sedation and weight gain. Adherence increased by 8% when patients were switched to divalproex ER.[16] Divalproex ER should also provide the clinician with easier and more reliable therapeutic drug monitoring. Similarly, an extended-release formulation of carbamazepine has been approved for the treatment of acute mania and a once-daily formulation of lithium is in development; these formulations should also theoretically improve adherence. However, differences in pharmacokinetics due to formulations may require dosage adjustments to achieve comparable serum concentrations and maintain efficacy. For example, converting a patient from divalproex DR to ER requires an increase in the total daily dose of 8% to 20% (i.e., divalproex DR 1,000 mg/day to divalproex ER 1,080 to 1,200 mg/day).[17]

Antipsychotics are also commonly used in the management of bipolar disorder, particularly during acute mania. The use of atypical antipsychotics, which are indicated for acute mania, acute bipolar depression, or maintenance, may improve adherence compared to typical antipsychotics. Similar to the situation in schizophrenia, the choice of which antipsychotic to use will depend on patient experience, patient preference, and the benefit–risk profiles of each respective agent. LAIs may also be used during the maintenance phase of treatment if adherence is an issue. The efficacy and safety of LAI risperidone were examined over 12 months in 11 stable patients with bipolar disorder who were switched from existing oral antipsychotic medication.[18] Most of the subjects (91%) completed the trial, and there were no significant changes in severity of symptoms or safety parameters. No subject reported a relapse when switched to LAI risperidone.[18]

Although this is controversial, antidepressants are frequently used in the treatment of bipolar depression. Optimization of antidepressant treatment, including simplification of the regimen and improved tolerability, for patients with bipolar disorder can be achieved through the use of novel formulations.

Stimulants

Stimulants are the cornerstone of therapy for patients with ADHD. While stimulants work extremely well, adherence can be problematic. Due to their short durations of action, multiple daily dosing is required for immediate-release formulations of stimulants to ensure adequate symptom control throughout the day. This reduces adherence because (1) inconsistent blood levels may not provide stable control of ADHD symptomatology; (2) peak-to-trough fluctuations in blood levels may result in increased side effects, including rebound phenomenon; (3) persons with ADHD may be more likely to forget to take their medications at multiple time points during the day due to the inherent nature of the disorder; and (4) there are practical issues, such as lack of privacy, with the administration of stimulants during the day, especially with children and adolescents (i.e., having to go to the nurse and being ridiculed by peers). To address these barriers to adherence, extended-release and transdermal preparations of stimulants have been developed. While the efficacy of these products is comparable to that of immediate-release formulations, the convenience and improved tolerability make extended-release and transdermal formulations preferred treatment options. With regard to symptom control, use of an extended-release formulation automatically lengthens the time these medications are actually treating symptoms of ADHD.

The market is flooded with a number of methylphenidate and amphetamine products in the following classes: immediate-release (4 to 6 hours of coverage), intermediate-acting (6 to 8 hours of coverage), and long-acting (10 to 12 hours of coverage). The use of long-acting preparations is considered the standard of care because of the extended coverage (i.e., school/work and afterwards). In addition, long-acting preparations have been shown to be associated with improved adherence,[19] which is important from the perspective of psychosocial functioning. Intermediate-acting preparations are generally used if coverage is required only during school/work hours. Immediate-release preparations can be used to supplement immediate- or long-acting stimulants if necessary (Table 5.4).

All stimulants have been found to equally effective for the management of ADHD.[19] The choice of what stimulant to use depends on several factors, including previous stimulant use and associated outcomes, coverage needed, tolerability, patient/parent preference, and cost.

A recent addition to the market is the methylphenidate transdermal system (MTS), which is applied once daily and delivers a consistent amount of methylphenidate during the time the patch is worn. MTS represents a useful option for

Table 5.4 Intermediate- and Long-Acting Stimulant Formulations

Drug/Formulation	Product	Characteristics	Duration of Effect (hours)/Daily Dosing
Dexmethylphenidate; extended release	Focalin XR	50% immediate release, 50% delayed release	10–12/once
Dextroamphetamine	Dexedrine Spansules	Bead with immediate and sustained release	4–9/multiple
Lisdexamfetamine	Vyvanse	Prodrug converted to dextroamphetamine	12/once
Methylphenidate; biphasic release	Concerta	22% immediate release, 78% delayed release	10–12/once
	Metadate CD	30% immediate release, 70% delayed release	8/once
	Ritalin LA	50% immediate release, 50% delayed release	6–8/once
Methylphenidate; sustained release	Metadate ER	Slow, continual release	4–8/multiple
	Methylin ER	Slow, continual release	4–8/multiple
	Ritalin SR	Slow, continual release	4–6/multiple
Methylphenidate; transdermal	Daytrana	Consistent release dependent on patch size and wear time	Wear time/once
Mixed amphetamine salts	Adderall XR	50% immediate release, 50% delayed release	10–12/once

patients who have difficultly swallowing or tolerating oral formulations, or for those who need or desire improved control of the duration of medication effect. The total dose delivered depends on patch size and wear time (over a 9-hour period: 10 mg for 27.5 mg patch, 15 mg for 41.3 mg patch, 20 mg for 55 mg patch, and 30 mg for 82.5mg patch).

Lisdexamfetamine, a prodrug stimulant that is converted to active dextroamphetamine after oral ingestion, was developed to provide an extended, consistent duration of effect with reduced potential for abuse and tampering and overdose toxicity. Because the pharmacokinetic profile of lisdexamfetamine depends on the prodrug, a formulation that extended the delivery is not necessary as seen with other stimulants. In addition, a smoother rise and consistent time to maximum plasma levels with lisdexamfetamine may provide for a more predictable response. These attributes could theoretically translate into improved patient adherence and outcomes.

Approximately a quarter of persons with ADHD will not respond to a stimulant or will have intolerable side effects.[19] Nonstimulant medications may be viable treatment options for these individuals. Bupropion and tricyclic antidepressants (desipramine, nortriptyline) are among the antidepressants studied for ADHD. Sustained- and extended-release formulations of bupropion may improve tolerability and adherence.[15] Alpha-agonist clonidine is available as a transdermal system, and an extended-release preparation of guanfacine is being developed. Atomoxetine is a long-acting norepinephrine reuptake inhibitor that is administered once daily, but the clinical effects take weeks for full onset.

Other psychotropic medications

Advances in formulations of medications have had a positive impact on factors that affect adherence in other psychiatric and neurologic disorders. In patients with alcohol dependence, injectable depot formulations of naltrexone have been shown to minimize the plasma fluctuations seen with oral naltrexone, resulting in uncompromised efficacy and reduced adverse effects. Depot naltrexone also offers convenience to patients.[20] Similarly, the introduction of a rivastigmine patch for patients with Alzheimer's disease may improve adherence. The rivastigmine patch has comparable efficacy to oral capsules but improved tolerability due to less fluctuating, more continuous drug delivery.[21] Caregivers of Alzheimer's patients expressed greater satisfaction with administration of the rivastigmine patch compared to capsules, and this may increase adherence.[22]

Formulations in development

The introduction of LAI risperidone to the market was a significant advancement with regard to the role of LAI antipsychotics for the clinical management of patients with schizophrenia. LAI formulations of other atypical antipsychotics are in various stages of development and testing. For example, a LAI formulation of olanzapine that sustains plasma olanzapine concentrations for over a month after a single injection has been developed and is under federal review. A paliperidone palmitate LAI formulation is also being developed with the aim of achieving sustained plasma levels over a 1-month period. It is possible that the technology used in these novel LAI formulations may allow for longer intervals, such as 3 months. Extended intervals for injection administration may improve adherence as it may be more convenient for patients. As seen with the oral formulations of atypical antipsychotics, clinicians will have options when additional LAI atypical antipsychotics become available on the market. Until systematic head-to-head comparisons are conducted, *the decision of which LAI antipsychotic medication to use should depend on the patient's past experiences with oral antipsychotics, the patient's preference (i.e., interval duration), an evaluation of benefits and risks, and availability/cost.*

Surgical implants represent the next line of formulations of psychotropic medications designed to improve medication adherence. Surgical implants provide patient autonomy over treatment, as patients can make long-term decisions about their pharmacological treatment. Surgical implants also provide more stable plasma concentrations, resulting in fewer adverse effects, and can be removed in lieu of a serious adverse effect. The use of surgical implants will require informed consent, and thus the patient will need to be in relatively good mental health.

Naltrexone implants, which are being developed and studied for the management of opioid addiction, are designed to provide 3 to 6 months of drug administration. In a postdetoxification study of 83 patients, naltrexone implants were shown to increase adherence and abstinence rates compared to oral naltrexone.[23] Although not yet tested in humans, the feasibility of surgical implants of haloperidol and risperidone has been examined in rodents.[24,25] Haloperidol implants provided a steady release of drug for 5 months, resulting in increased striatal dopamine-2 receptor expression.[24] Risperidone implants showed drug release for 2 months or more.[25]

Pharmacogenetics

Without question, the future of medicine is personalized prescription through pharmacogenetics. As seen in other fields of medicine, pharmacogenetics can be used to select and tailor pharmacological treatment regimens based on genetic variance. For example, trastuzumab treatment for breast cancer requires pharmacogenetic testing of humanized anti-human epidermal growth factor receptor type 2 (HER2) expression and gene amplification, as increasing evidence suggests clinical benefit in patients who show overexpression or amplification of HER2. Similarly, the field of psychiatry can benefit tremendously from pharmacogenetic testing to maximize treatment response and minimize safety and tolerability problems. This is relevant in the context of medication adherence as lack of response and poor tolerability are among the common reasons for medication discontinuation in patients with psychiatric illnesses.

Pharmacogenetic testing in clinical practice

Although limited, testing of genes affecting pharmacokinetics is available and being used in clinical psychiatric practice. Cytochrome P450 (CYP) genotype testing has been incorporated in psychiatric hospitals and clinics across the nation. Specifically, assessments of two polymorphic genes, the cytochrome P450 2D6 (CYP2D6) and 2C19 (CYP2C19), using the FDA-approved AmpliChip CYP450 Test have been conducted.[26] CYP2D6 is involved in the metabolism of antidepressants and antipsychotics, and CYP2C19 is involved in the metabolism of antidepressants (Table 5.5).

Certain variants in these polymorphic genes confer differential effectiveness of drug metabolism (Fig. 5.2). For CYP2D6, patients are characterized as poor metabolizers (PM), intermediate metabolizers (IM), extensive metabolizers (EM), or ultra-rapid metabolizers (UM).[26] For CYP2C19, patients are either EMs or PMs.[26] Ethnic variation in genotype distributions is present, with 5% to 10% of Caucasians being CYP2D6 PMs, 10% to 29% of North Africans and Middle Easterners being CYP2D6 UMs, and 10% to 25% of East Asians being CYP2C19 PMs.[26] In practice settings where CYP genotype testing is not readily available or feasible to due to cost, prediction of drug metabolism can possibly be based on ethnicity (Table 5.6).

Knowledge of a patient's CYP genotype can be very helpful throughout the course of treatment. Metabolizer status can significantly affect plasma concentrations of psychotropic medications, which in turn can be related

Table 5.5 Psychotropic Substrates of CYP2D6 and CYP2C19

CYP2D6	CYP2C19
Antipsychotics	**Antidepressants**
Aripiprazole	Citalopram
Fluphenazine	Clomipramine
Haloperidol	Escitalopram
Perphenazine	Imipramine
Risperidone	Sertraline
Thioridazine	
Antidepressants	
Amitriptyline	
Amoxapine	
Clomipramine	
Desipramine	
Doxepin	
Duloxetine	
Fluoxetine	
Fluvoxamine	
Imipramine	
Mirtazpine	
Nortriptyline	
Paroxetine	
Venlafaxine	

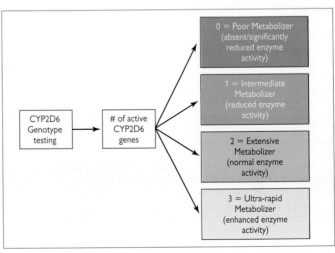

Figure 5.2 CYP2D6 genotypes and phenotypes.

Table 5.6 Summary of CYP2D6 and CYP2C19 Phenotypes and Clinical Implications

Phenotype	2D6	2C19	Clinical Implications
Poor metabolizer (PM)	Yes	Yes	• Increased risk of side effects due to elevated concentrations of active drug
Intermediate metabolizer (IM)	Yes		• May increased risk of side effects due to elevated concentrations of active drug • May reduced response if prodrug is minimally or not metabolized at all
Extensive metabolizer (EM)	Yes	Yes	• Expected response to standard doses
Ultra-rapid metabolizer (UM)	Yes		• Nonresponse due to reduced concentrations of active drug • Increased risk of side effects due to elevated concentrations of active metabolite • May seem like nonadherence due to reduced concentrations of active drug

to treatment effectiveness and susceptibility to adverse drug reactions. Poor metabolism likely results in high plasma concentrations of the active parent compound and an increased risk of adverse effects. In a large naturalistic study, Grasmader and colleagues[27] found increased plasma levels of various antidepressants and associated side effects in depressed inpatients who were characterized as CYP2D6 PMs. Poor metabolism of antipsychotics has also been related to an increased risk of extrapyramidal symptoms (EPS) and QTc prolongation. de Leon and colleagues[28] reported that PMs of risperidone had a threefold increase in the odds of moderate to severe adverse effects, most of which were EPS. Thioridazine plasma concentrations have been shown to be increased in individuals with poor CYP2D6 enzyme activity, which may confer a greater risk of QTc prolongation and cardiotoxicity.[29] In fact, thioridazine is contraindicated with people that are known to have a genetic defect leading to reduced levels of activity of P450 2D6 isoenzyme. Thus, standard dosing of psychotropic medications may not be appropriate for PMs, and clinicians should consider using lower doses (30% to 70% reduction from standard dose) or alternative agents that are not metabolized by CYP2D6 or CYP2C19.[30] Poor metabolizer status may also affect the therapeutic response if the administered agent is a prodrug and requires biotransformation to an active metabolite. However, there are currently no psychotropic agents that require CYP2D6 or CYP2C19 for pharmacological activity.[30]

Relative to poor metabolism, the clinical significance of ultra-rapid metabolism is not as much understood. CYP2D6 ultra-rapid metabolism likely results in subtherapeutic plasma concentrations of medications at standard doses;[26,30] possible consequences may be poor response and increased metabolite-related side effects. For UMs, dose increases of 135% to 180% or the use of alternative agents not metabolized through CYP2D6 has been recommended.[30] In the context of medication adherence, a patient who is an UM may seem as if he or she is nonadherent to the CYP2D6 dependent antidepressant or antipsychotic.

Because polypharmacy is quite prevalent in psychiatry, clinicians need to keep in mind that a number of psychotropic medications are powerful inhibitors and inducers of the CYP450 isoenzyme system. Coadministration of one of these particular agents may change a patient's metabolizer status. For example, an EM taking fluoxetine, which is a CYP2D6 inhibitor, may present like a PM. One half to two thirds of CYP2D6 EMs taking standard doses of fluoxetine, paroxetine, or bupropion present like PMs.[31]

Progress in pharmacogenetic testing

Genotype testing for additional candidate genes affecting the pharmacokinetics or pharmacodynamics of psychotropic medications is currently limited to research efforts. While the clinical relevance of these polymorphisms needs further investigation, the utility of such genotype testing may eventually be realized in the context of personalized prescription in clinical psychiatric practice (Table 5.7).

Table 5.7 Selected Candidate Genes and Possible Clinical Relevance[32–38]		
Gene	**Drug(s)**	**Possible clinical relevance**
Pharmacokinetics		
ABCB1	Antidepressants	• Pharmacokinetics (SSRIs)
	Methadone	• Dose requirements
Pharmacodynamics		
5HT1A receptor	Antipsychotics	• Response (negative and depressive symptoms)
5HT2A receptor	Antidepressants	• Response
	Antipsychotics	• Response (clozapine)
		• Risk of tardive dyskinesia
5HT2C receptor	Antipsychotics	• Response (clozapine)
		• Risk of tardive dyskinesia
		• Weight gain
5HTTLPR	Antidepressants	• Response (SSRIs)
		• Adverse effects (SSRIs)
		• Antidepressant-induced mania
ABCB1	Antidepressants	• Response (P-gp substrates)
ADRA2A	Stimulants	• Response (methylphenidate)
BDNF	Antidepressants	• Response
	Antipsychotics	• Response (clozapine)
		• Risk of extrapyramidal symptoms
COMT	Stimulants	• Response (methylphenidate)
CREB1	Antidepressants	• Treatment-emergent suicidal ideation
DAT1	Stimulants	• Response (methylphenidate)
DRD2	Antipsychotics	• Response (clozapine, risperidone)
DRD3	Antipsychotics	• Response
		• Risk of tardive dyskinesia
DRD4	Antipsychotics	• Response (clozapine)
	Stimulants	• Response (methylphenidate)
FKBP5	Antidepressants	• Response
GRIA3	Antidepressants	• Treatment-emergent suicidal ideation
GRIK2	Antidepressants	• Treatment-emergent suicidal ideation
GRIK4	Antidepressants	• Response (SSRIs)
SNAP-25	Antipsychotics	• Weight gain

References

1. Eldred LJ, Wu AW, Chaisson RE, Moore RD. Adherence to antiretroviral and pneumocystis prophylaxis in HIV disease. *J Acquir Immune Defic Syndr Hum Retrovirol.* 1998;18:117–125.

2. Iskedjian M, Einarson TR, MacKeigan LD, et al. Relationship between daily dose frequency and adherence to antihypertensive pharmacotherapy: evidence from a meta-analysis. *Clin Ther.* 2002;24:302–316.

3. Melikian C, White TJ, Vanderplas A, Dezii CM, Chang E. Adherence to oral antidiabetic therapy in a managed care organization: a comparison of mono-therapy, combination therapy, and fixed-dose combination therapy. *Clin Ther.* 2002;24:460–467.

4. Dolder CR, Lacro JP, Dunn LB, Jeste DV. Antipsychotic medication adherence: is there a difference between typical and atypical agents? *Am J Psychiatry.* 2002;159:103–108.

5. Valenstein M, Blow FC, Copeland LA, et al. Poor antipsychotic adherence among patients with schizophrenia: medication and patient factors. *Schizophr Bull.* 2004;30:255–264.

6. Lieberman JA, Stroup TS, McEvoy JP, et al. Effectiveness of antipsychotic drugs in patients with chronic schizophrenia. *N Engl J Med.* 2005;353: 1209–1223.

7. Lacro JP, Dunn LB, Dolder CR, Leckband SG, Jeste DV. Prevalence of and risk factors for medication nonadherence in patients with schizophrenia: a comprehensive review of recent literature. *J Clin Psychiatry.* 2002;63:892–909.

8. Chengappa KN, Parepally H, Brar JS, Mullen J, Shilling A, Goldstein JM. A random-assignment, double-blind, clinical trial of once- vs twice-daily administration of quetiapine fumarate in patients with schizophrenia or schizoaffective disorder: a pilot study. *Can J Psychiatry.* 2003;48:187–194.

9. Ganesan S, Agambaram V, Randeree F, Eggens I, Huizar K, Meulien D. Switching from other antipsychotics to once-daily extended release quetiapine fumarate in patients with schizophrenia. *Curr Med Res Opin.* 2008;24:21–32.

10. Keith S. Advances in psychotropic formulations. *Prog Neuropsychopharmacol Biol Psychiatry.* 2006;30:996–1008.

11. Schooler NR. Relapse and rehospitalization: comparing oral and depot antipsychotics. *J Clin Psychiatry.* 2003;64(Suppl 16):14–17.

12. Adams CE, Fenton MK, Quraishi S, David AS. Systematic meta-review of depot antipsychotic drugs for people with schizophrenia. *Br J Psychiatry.* 2001;179:290–299.

13. Glazer WM, Kane JM. Depot neuroleptic therapy: an underutilized treatment option. *J Clin Psychiatry.* 1992;53:426–433.

14. Walburn J, Gray R, Gournay K, Quraishi S, David AS. Systematic review of patient and nurse attitudes to depot antipsychotic medication. *Br J Psychiatry.* 2001;179:300–307.

15. Fava M, Rush AJ, Thase ME, et al. 15 years of clinical experience with bupropion HCl: from bupropion to bupropion SR to bupropion XL. *Prim Care Companion J Clin Psychiatry.* 2005;7:106–113.

16. Minirth FB, Neal V. Assessment of patient preference and side effects in patients switched from divalproex sodium delayed release to divalproex sodium extended release. *J Clin Psychopharmacol.* 2005;25:99–101.

17. Dutta S, Reed RC. Divalproex to divalproex extended release conversion. *Clin Drug Investig.* 2004;24:495–508.

18. Han C, Lee MS, Pae CU, Ko YH, Patkar AA, Jung IK. Usefulness of long-acting injectable risperidone during 12-month maintenance therapy of bipolar disorder. *Prog Neuropsychopharmacol Biol Psychiatry.* 2007;31:1219–1223.

19. Connor DF, Meltzer BM. *Pediatric Psychopharmacology Fast Facts.* New York: W.W. Norton & Company, Inc.; 2006.

20. Johnson BA. Naltrexone long-acting formulation in the treatment of alcohol dependence. *Ther Clin Risk Manag.* 2007;3:741–749.

21. Winblad B, Grossberg G, Frolich L, et al. IDEAL: a 6-month, double-blind, placebo-controlled study of the first skin patch for Alzheimer disease. *Neurology.* 2007;69:S14–22.

22. Winblad B, Kawata AK, Beusterien KM, et al. Caregiver preference for rivastigmine patch relative to capsules for treatment of probable Alzheimer's disease. *Int J Geriatr Psychiatry.* 2007;22:485–491.

23. Colquhoun R, Tan DY, Hull S. A comparison of oral and implant naltrexone outcomes at 12 months. *J Opioid Manag.* 2005;1:249–256.

24. Siegel SJ, Winey KI, Gur RE, et al. Surgically implantable long-term antipsychotic delivery systems for the treatment of schizophrenia. *Neuropsychopharmacology.* 2002;26:817–823.

25. Rabin C, Liang Y, Ehrlichman RS, et al. In vitro and in vivo demonstration of risperidone implants in mice. *Schizophr Res.* 2008;98:66–78.

26. de Leon J, Armstrong SC, Cozza KL. Clinical guidelines for psychiatrists for the use of pharmacogenetic testing for CYP450 2D6 and CYP450 2C19. *Psychosomatics.* 2006;47:75–85.

27. Grasmader K, Verwohlt PL, Rietschel M, et al. Impact of polymorphisms of cytochrome-P450 isoenzymes 2C9, 2C19 and 2D6 on plasma concentrations and clinical effects of antidepressants in a naturalistic clinical setting. *Eur J Clin Pharmacol.* 2004;60:329–336.

28. de Leon J, Susce MT, Pan RM, Fairchild M, Koch WH, Wedlund PJ. The CYP2D6 poor metabolizer phenotype may be associated with risperidone adverse drug reactions and discontinuation. *J Clin Psychiatry.* 2005;66:15–27.

29. A LL, Berecz R, de la Rubia A, Dorado P. QTc interval lengthening is related to CYP2D6 hydroxylation capacity and plasma concentration of thioridazine in patients. *J Psychopharmacol.* 2002;16:361–364.

30. Maier W, Zobel A. Contribution of allelic variations to the phenotype of response to antidepressants and antipsychotics. *Eur Arch Psychiatry Clin Neurosci.* 2008;258(Suppl 1):12–20.

31. Alfaro CL, Lam YW, Simpson J, Ereshefsky L. CYP2D6 status of extensive metabolizers after multiple-dose fluoxetine, fluvoxamine, paroxetine, or sertraline. *J Clin Psychopharmacol.* 1999;19:155–163.

32. Abdolmaleky HM, Thiagalingam S, Wilcox M. Genetics and epigenetics in major psychiatric disorders: dilemmas, achievements, applications, and future scope. *Am J Pharmacogenomics.* 2005;5:149–160.

33. Foster A, Miller del D, Buckley PF. Pharmacogenetics and schizophrenia. *Psychiatr Clin North Am.* 2007;30:417–435.

34. Reynolds GP. The impact of pharmacogenetics on the development and use of antipsychotic drugs. *Drug Discov Today.* 2007;12:953–959.

35. Lin E, Chen PS. Pharmacogenomics with antidepressants in the STAR*D study. *Pharmacogenomics.* 2008;9:935–946.

36. Serretti A, Artioli P. The pharmacogenomics of selective serotonin reuptake inhibitors. *Pharmacogenomics J.* 2004;4:233–244.

37. Faraone SV, Khan SA. Candidate gene studies of attention-deficit hyperactivity disorder. *J Clin Psychiatry.* 2006;67(Suppl 8):13–20.

38. Somogyi AA, Barratt DT, Coller JK. Pharmacogenetics of opioids. *Clin Pharmacol Ther.* 2007;81:429–444.

Chapter 6

Nonpharmacological options for managing nonadherence

Assessment of medication adherence is inconsistent even in clinical drug trials, with only 19% of clinical trials measuring drug adherence in 1974 and up to 47% in 1997–1999.[1] Although research data on nonadherence are mounting (Chapters 2, 3, and 4), adherence assessment in clinicians' offices is inconsistent and adherence is rarely measured formally. Those who pursue measuring, monitoring, and understanding treatment nonadherence encounter complex issues that may involve changes in personal attitudes and beliefs and acute awareness of their own countertransference, stereotypes, and cultural and scientific biases. When preparing this book, we asked mental health services consumers in Georgia, in the United States, to give us their input on the topic of adherence. Some of the responses we received are included in this chapter, and we are particularly grateful for their insights into this issue. Before presenting the findings from literature on the psychosocial methods that enhance medication adherence in psychiatric illnesses, we will go over basic issues that are at the core of understanding these nonpharmacological measures and could help clinicians develop their own adherence "toolkit."

The basics

Assess and monitor nonadherence

With no-show rates for the initial psychiatric appointment around 25% and rates for follow-up appointments of 15% to 40% (Chapter 2), psychiatrists deal with missed appointments as an objective manifestation of nonadherence. Recording missed appointments, communicating clearly about expectation to keep appointments, obtaining and offering adequate contact information, discussing reasons for missed appointments, and reminding patients that mental health treatment is the tool they chose to solve emotional problems can all help reduce no-show rates. Once the patient is in the office, one can integrate adherence rating scales or other adherence assessment methods in daily practice (Chapter 4 and Adherence Toolkit).

"What is the range and the average time people spend with a psychiatrist?"

—J. Rock

Allow patients to talk spontaneously

The average patient visiting a family practice office in the United States talks only 23 seconds before the doctor takes the lead. While these data come from outside the psychiatric field, this likely represents a trend across specialties under present practice conditions. A German study allowed patients to talk uninterrupted at the first office contact with their internists. The mean spontaneous talking time was 92 seconds, and almost 80% of people finished their initial report in less than 2 minutes.[2] This suggests that allowing patients to give information without interrupting them is not too time-consuming and can be a tool to engage and gain the patient's trust.

> *"One reason I think people don't take medication as prescribed is a belief that the psychiatrist wasn't listening to them, didn't hear them and, consequently, is not prepared to appropriately subscribe."*
>
> — J. Rock

> *"MH [mental health] professionals need to question themselves as to what they contribute to people not taking their meds. This is a two-way problem, not the unitary responsibility of the 'nonadherent patient' whose behavior needs to be fixed."*
>
> — J. Rock

Form a therapeutic alliance

Psychiatrists' ability to "develop and maintain a therapeutic alliance with patients by instilling feelings of trust, honesty, openness, rapport, and comfort in the relationship with physicians" is a core competency for our specialty.[3] The therapeutic alliance has been repeatedly linked with beneficial outcomes and, when combined with effective treatment modalities, is at the root of treatment success. Patients' nonadherence frequently involves issues of the therapeutic alliance. Also, an alliance that exists when people are treatment-adherent may quickly dissolve in the presence of an illness relapse caused by nonadherence. As dual treatment, where a psychiatrist and psychotherapist both provide mental health care to same patient, becomes widespread and the duration of the medication management visit shrinks, the therapeutic relationship with the mentally ill risks erosion. In fact, integrated treatment by the same provider has been proven to yield higher medication adherence[4] and to be more cost-effective than dual treatment. As consumers' perspectives about psychotropic medication are now being heard, the terms used to describe patients' involvement in their own treatment evolve, and so does our understanding of the underpinnings of adherence (see Chapter 1, Table 1.4).

Among the building blocks of the therapeutic relationship are the patient's perception of the potential risks and benefits of the treatment, the physician's judgment of the same (Chapter 3), and the beliefs, emotions, and expectations that the patient and mental health professional bring to the relationship, otherwise known as transference and countertransference.

Transference can be idealizing—the belief that the psychopharmacologist has a "magic pill." If the medication somehow fails, splitting and anger toward the psychopharmacologist may ensue, while the patient complains only to the therapist. Splitting can be accentuated by the very nature of the dual treatment, with demands on the patient to discuss all medication issues with the pharmacologist while saving all the emotional issues for the therapist. Narcissistic injury, gratitude, and passive acceptance can all occur in response to prescribing medication. Delving into patients' experience and attitudes about medication can be an important tool in understanding their inner life, including their ego functioning, relationships, and defenses. Thus, a thorough review of the dynamics, transference, and countertransference should be included in each "medication-refractory" patient evaluation.[4]

Countertransference in face of treatment nonadherence is a common and ego-threatening occurrence, especially for physicians. Countertransference is often experienced as disappointment, anger, hopelessness, distancing, and ultimately blame directed toward the patient. In the presence of a dependent patient one can develop rescue fantasies and become overinvolved. If the provider can recognize these responses, he or she can address them, take responsibility to improve the therapeutic relationship, and re-evaluate the treatment plan, holding the patient's point of view at high regard.[3]

Beyond transference, patients' cultural and spiritual beliefs, as well as fear of devaluation of self-agency by interfering with their control of their life and goals, are likely to color patients' experience with medication. Delving into those issues may help us find ways to address and improve treatment adherence. Deegan[5] offers a new perspective on pharmacological treatment when she describes the medication compliance model as simplistic and introduces the concept of "personal medicine defined as non-pharmaceutical, self-initiated activities that serve to decrease symptoms, avoid undesirable outcomes and improve well being." A study on a shared decision-making tool that patients complete and hand to the provider at each outpatient visit showed promising preliminary results. The tool elicits a symptomatic and functional inventory, assesses medication-related concerns and goals, and reminds severely mentally ill patients of their "personal medicine."

The *psychiatric advance directive (PAD)* is a relatively new health services approach in psychiatry: only 3% to 14% of outpatients in public mental health system use advance directives. The directive allows patients to decide which treatment they would prefer to have in the case of an illness relapse during which they become incompetent. Although this is seen by some practitioners as a tool to refuse all psychiatric treatment even in cases when such behavior can lead to dangerousness, research shows that directives have the potential to improve patients' working alliance with their clinicians and are generally used by patients to express preferences about facilities where they would not want to be hospitalized and medications they do or do not want to take. Cases where people use the psychiatric advance directives to refuse all treatment are rare.

Treatment education

Some patients' condition may improve if they know their diagnosis and have positive expectations of response to the treatment given. Particular regions of the brain have been implicated in the placebo response in treatment of depression. One week after treatment was started, depressed patients taking either fluoxetine or placebo had regional metabolic changes on fluoro-deoxy-glucose positive emission tomography in the ventral striatal and orbital frontal areas of the brain, before any clinical improvement occurred. These functional changes predicted which patients ultimately responded to fluoxetine after 6 weeks of treatment and did not occur in nonresponders. When patients respond to antidepressants clinically, different areas in the brain show metabolic changes, namely the hippocampus, brain stem, and posterior cingulate gyrus, pointing to a specific effect of "reward expectation" on the brain.[6] Another aspect of education involves "normalizing" treatment options offered to patients by placing them in context of treatment algorithms, presenting data about the frequency and efficacy of their use, especially with medications like MAO inhibitors, clozapine, LAI antipsychotics (Chapter 5), somatic treatments like electroconvulsive therapy (ECT), vagal nerve stimulation, transcranial magnetic stimulation and intensive psychosocial methods like assertive community treatment (ACT). Presenting explicitly to the ECT candidate that this method is used at a rate of 140 treatments per 100,000 population and 77% of patients who received ECT thought 4 years later that ECT was at least satisfactory if not excellent or even life-saving may reduce stigma or at least open the door for questions from the patient. Psychoeducation, however, has limited effect on adherence when applied alone in chronic, severe mental illness, as described later in this chapter.

> "When I tried to tell not one, not even just two, but at least three different people that [drug x] made me…see a violent red wash over my eyes and make me want to physically harm [anyone]……How did those I approached react to my heartened plea for feedback…? 'That medicine doesn't do that to anyone.'"
>
> —Cindy Sue Causey

> "A lot of the meds have side effects dealing with sun exposure, constipation, lactation, uncontrollable tremors, 'sleep eating,' sleep problems (too little/much), the 'shuffle,' all of the mainstream side effects that most people share. Being introduced to new medications is sort of like walking around in a dark room without shoes: sooner or later, I'm going to find something unpleasant to bump into. I used to think that I was a fairly compliant patient, but after many, MANY reaction processes over the years, I have grown to be hesitant about the meds, and at times resistant."
>
> —Alison

> "Psychiatrists don't explain why they choose medications, nor do they discuss adequately 'side effects' or serious signs to watch for, rash for example."
>
> —J. Rock

Listen to adverse events; individualize each patient's treatment

The consumer quotes listed above prompts one to wonder if these people have a polymorphism of glutamate receptor genes found to be associated with treatment-emergent suicidal ideation or have a CYP450 enzyme polymorphism (Chapter 5). Considering the advancement of pharmacogenetics (Chapter 5), it is fair to say that approximately 5% of Caucasians who are poor metabolizers of CYP2D6 may not be able to tolerate average doses of a common antidepressant like venlafaxine or an antipsychotic like risperidone; this proportion may be even higher than 5% if we add the patients on polypharmacy regimens, where certain drugs act as metabolic enzyme inhibitors and could slow down the metabolism of enzyme substrates, thus creating a potentially harmful effect. In these cases, 100% adherence with treatment may not be an option. There are challenges in adopting existing pharmacogenetic knowledge: although the tests available to date help us better appreciate a patient's risk in taking a particular medication, they do not predict outcome; they are expensive and we do not know if they are cost-effective. On the other hand, people who experience adverse effects early in treatment are more likely to be nonadherent with treatment later. Using results of pharmacogenetic tests to avoid adverse effects at first contact with medication and to individualize doses to avoid future side effects may improve alliance and adherence to medication and thus may be worth pursuing.

> "I wish somebody would do the research on how long-term use of medications affect the body and brain, as well as what nutritional supplements might help ameliorate symptoms and negative side effects. When I take all three as prescribed by the psychiatrist, my holistic kinesiologist nutritionist says that my liver needs support to metabolize and detox the drugs, and recommends a bunch of different supplements and herbs. However, when I

don't take them, he recommends only a few basic supplements. Therefore, I feel that taking the drugs has a negative effect on my health, which makes me want to discontinue use."

—Anonymous

Alternative medicine and nutrition

In 2000, of over 9,000 people surveyed, 16.5% used CAM, defined as homeopathy, acupuncture, massage therapy, herbal products, and spiritual healing. Over 21% of the responders were diagnosed with mental illness, and of those, people with panic and major depression were more likely to use alternative medicine. "Conventional" mental health providers face a tidal wave of complementary therapies and the need to integrate them into the treatment plan while encouraging or preserving adherence to conventional therapies. Frequent reviews of literature or use of computerized drug interaction computer software programs that include herbal products can be critical to maintain safe prescribing to patients who also use CAM and at the same time to validate patients' involvement with such treatment tools. The National Center for Complementary and Alternative Medicine's Web site (http://nccam.nih.gov/) offers research on mental health topics and scientific support for various therapies. Various institutions support centers that combine conventional and alternative medicine and have staff specialized in the application of integrative approaches to mental health, such as the University of California San Francisco Osher Center for Integrative Medicine (http://www.osher.ucsf.edu/), Duke Integrative Medicine (www.dukeintegrativemedicine.org), and the Jefferson Myrna Brind Center of Integrative Medicine (http://jeffline.jefferson.edu/JMBCIM/). The burden falls on us to remain current on this topic, although the integration of this aspect of psychopharmacology is just now starting to penetrate in medical schools, residency training programs, and continuing education programs.

"What about the cooperation, or not, with a primary care doctor, who may or may not exist, about coordinating lab tests, especially as we drop dead in our late 50s from preventable disorders? And who is doing the work re: role of antipsychotics here?"

—J. Rock

Foster a relationship with primary care providers

In 2007, Mental Health America, a large U.S. nonprofit organization aiming to helping people live mentally healthier lives, surveyed a sample of 250 adults with schizophrenia and 250 psychiatrists about their perspective on overall health care in mental health settings. Forty-four percent of all respondents reported being obese and 23% had diabetes. Psychiatrists reported discussing general health issues, but the vast majority of them felt that lack of time or not being as well equipped as primary care physicians to address patients' overall health prevented them from providing overall care. In turn, the majority of patients felt that treatment of their overall health, not just their mental illness, is essential to their recovery. The survey came in the wake of the finding by the U.S. National Association of State Mental Health Program Directors that people with serious mental illness are now dying 25 years earlier than the general population and their call for integration of mental and physical health care.

Despite such warning signs, the delineation of the responsibility of primary care physicians and psychiatrists in monitoring treatment adverse effects and the overall well-being of severely mentally ill people is not clear. While struggling with time limitations for patient visits, reimbursement cuts, and office staff limitations, psychiatrists are faced with the need to adhere to current monitoring guidelines for second-generation antipsychotics (vital signs, weight, waist circumference, and signs of hyperglycemia and hyperlipidemia) or, in the case of schizophrenia, broader health monitoring, including periodic assessment of motivation for smoking cessation, high-risk behaviors for HIV or hepatitis, immunization status, safety at home, and health habits in general (Table 6.1).[7]

Although many patients are now taking second-generation antipsychotics, the minority of people still on first-generation antipsychotics need to be monitored for movement adverse effects. Similarly, treatment of people with bipolar disorder often requires simultaneous treatment of comorbid conditions: migraine, pain disorders, cardiovascular disease, diabetes and obesity, therapeutic drug monitoring of mood stabilizer agents, and heightened awareness for potential additional effects from polypharmacy, which may in turn require additional treatment. In any condition, the simple gesture of making a phone contact with another provider in the patient's presence can solidify the therapeutic alliance, while the patient's response to such act may offer important information.[4]

> *"There are various devices that give notice of time for pill-taking; perhaps they can be researched and discussed, including Blackberry. Maybe the American Psychiatric Association could establish a scholarship fund for such devices; Medicaid will not pay for them. Also I know someone whose only CMHS service and at their request is to get a call to remind them to take their meds."*
>
> —J. Rock

Medication reminders: devices and interventions

A wide variety of medication reminder devices are available for purchase, such as a pill box and reminder system that automatically dispenses medication in accordance with prescription (http://www.assistedliving-store.com/p-30-medtime-xl-pill-box-reminder.aspx) and a stop watch with countdown and elapsed timer application for a Blackberry device (http://www.clickapps.com/moreinfo.htm?pid=8038&section=RIM). A computerized reminder device, the Disease Management Assistance System, which issues prerecorded timed messages, was shown to increase adherence in patients with HIV taking HAART, although the ratings on the quality-of-life scale decreased in the group that used the electronic reminder. A daily telephone call as well as a daily videotelephone call reminder yielded better results on medication adherence in elderly patients than no reminder at all. Some interventions, for example the MEMOPATCH, a dermal patch with a pulse generator that gives the patient a perceptible stimulus to the skin as a reminder to take medication, could overcome the possible stigma that a person may experience using audible medication reminders in public places.

Velligan[8] pioneered research on environmental supports to improve adherence with treatment in schizophrenia and thus developed cognitive adaptation training (CAT), a psychosocial intervention using environmental supports such as signs, alarms, and checklists to cue and sequence adaptive behavior in the patient's home environment and ultimately enhance functioning. Both CAT and a variant focused on medication and appointment adherence (Pharm CAT) were proven to be superior to standard treatment of patients with schizophrenia in improving medication adherence. This treatment targets adherence to medication, medication education, and orientation for patients with schizophrenia. In an ongoing study, Pharm CAT is compared with standard treatment and the use of the Med-eMonitor™, an electronic device that holds up to 1 month's supply of up to five medications and is capable of cueing taking of medication, warning patients when they are taking the wrong medication or taking it at the wrong time, recording side effect complaints, and through modem hookup promptly alerting treatment staff of failure to take medication as prescribed.

Table 6.1 Guidelines for medical management of patients with schizophrenia

	Special Circumstances
Initial evaluation:	Starting Atypical Antipsychotics:
Medical history • Weight, height, BMI, BP, pulse • Assess risk behaviors, educate on disease prevention • Records and contact with primary care provider	• Baseline: Record BMI, waist circumference, BP, fasting glucose, fasting lipid profile • Weight/BMI: every 4 wks for 12 wks, then annually • BP, fasting glucose: repeat at 12 wks, then annually • Lipids: repeat at 12 wks, then every 5 years
Every visit:	Overweight patients:
• Review symptoms, medication changes and adherence • Review risk behaviors • Encourage smoking cessation	• Nutritional counseling, weight reduction program • Consider a weight-neutral antipsychoticw
Every 6 months:	Abnormal fasting glucose:
• Communicate with primary care physician • Assess records of weight, height, BMI, BP, pulse • Psychoeducational counseling as appropriate	• Nutritional counseling, exercise program • Medical assessment • Educate patient and caregiver on diabetes • Consider medication switch
Annually:	Smokers:
• Fasting glucose, BP • Confirm completion of annual screens (mammography, colonoscopy, pap smear), immunizations, health habits • Review residential safety • Set goals to enhance health	• Assess willingness to quit • Offer cessation advice, support, referrals • Frequent contact
	Hypertension:
	• Nutritional counseling, exercise program • Review salt intake, alcohol intake, diet • Encourage smoking cessation if needed • Refer for medical evaluation
	Hyperlipidemia:
	• Nutritional counseling, exercise program • Refer for medical evaluation, yearly lipid profiles • Consider medication switch
	High risk behavior:
	• Intensive behavioral education program • Counseling and HIV or hepatitis screens, as needed

(Adapted from Goff DC et al, J Clin Psychiatry 2005[7])

Be aware of involuntary commitment laws

In 1995, 35 U.S. states had outpatient commitment laws, and after a man with untreated schizophrenia pushed Kendra Webdale in front of an onpcoming sub-way train in New York City in 1999, more states developed such laws. Kendra's Law in New York and similar legislation in other states are meant to prevent de-compensation of people who have previously been hospitalized or incarcerated multiple times because of nonadherence with treatment for mental illness.[9] Such laws often do not authorize involuntary medication administration. After 5 years of having such a law in place in New York State, 6-month outcomes showed a significant drop in arrests, incarceration, psychiatric hospitalization, and home-lessness in over 2,700 people whose treatment included outpatient commitment. However, there was no control group for comparison, and New York State allo-cated additional funding for mental health services while the law was in force.[9]

In Australia, mandated psychiatric care is provided through community treat-ment orders. A controlled study on outcomes of the community treatment order showed that such treatment did not reduce hospitalization rates.[10]

Fear of forced treatment (involuntary hospitalization or forced medication) has been identified as a barrier to mental health treatment, especially by people who experienced mandated treatment in the past. The debate is ongoing as to whether outpatient commitment raises additional barriers that may negatively affect the therapeutic alliance or whether its enactment brings substantial benefit to a difficult-to-treat patient population.

Stay abreast of the recovery movement

Resilience, self-agency, and empowerment throughout all stages of illness are concepts emphasized by the consumer literature on recovery in mental illness. Resilience is defined as the "capacity to adapt, cope, rebound, withstand, grow, survive, and define a new self through adversity."[5] Academicians have tried to articulate a clinical definition of recovery, concluding it to be symptom remission for at least 2 years along with satisfactory vocational functioning, independent living, and peer relationships. However, consumers have a much broader view of recovery that encompasses their life journey: recovery is viewed more as a process than as an outcome. People in recovery prefer to view their illness in terms of a condition that they need to cope with and integrate into their world experience, rather than be defined by it. Recovery is a journey of healing. People recovering seek the support of others who have similar experiences to help guide them through their situation.

The peer support specialist notion is derived partially from AA. A peer sup-port specialist is a person pursuing his or her own recovery who has also received specific training to equip him or her to contribute to the care of other persons. The U.S. Substance Abuse and Mental Health Services Administration and other agencies are providing funding to demonstrate this concept around the United States with the Certified Peer Specialist Project. The project places peer spe-cialists in community mental health centers, in assertive community treatment teams, at VA hospitals, and in medical schools. Involvement in consumer-operat-ed services may positively affect various dimensions of recovery.[11] Psychiatrists' own reports of recovery-oriented practices show that while psychiatrists aware of recovery practices frequently asked about their patients' social situation, hous-ing, work and life goals, they did not always endorse peer support, make contact with families, or seek to change a patient's environment. Recovery awareness may be associated with less authoritarian medication management by psychia-trists. Finding the balance between recovery principles and, when necessary, application of authoritarian methods of treatment (involuntary hospitalization and outpatient commitment) appears to be a challenge for psychiatrists. The relationship between the provider's adherence to recovery principles and the patient's treatment adherence has not yet been explored; it appears that applying these principles could improve trust and alliance between people with mental illness and their providers. Accordingly, peer support specialists might be able to provide more first-hand experience, including how medication felt to them, whether it worked or not, and what side effects to look out for. A peer support specialist might deintensify the experience of taking medication and might offer hope and support to the other person. On the other hand, some peer support specialists believe less in medication, and some (perhaps many) have had bad previous experiences with medication. Sharing these viewpoints and experiences could also influence whether the person takes his or her medication or not.

Include motivational interviewing and cognitive–behavioral and interpersonal therapy in routine medication management visits

Elements of cognitive–behavioral therapy (CBT) may be applicable in routine medication management sessions or case manager encounters and have been researched in severe mental illness; thus, familiarity with these principles may benefit any clinician.[12,13]

Motivational approaches to treatment are extensively used to engage and maintain people in treatment of substance use disorders[14] and are designed to enhance one's internal motivation to change. Brief motivational interventions can be delivered in single sessions. Motivational interviewing is a technique based on the stages of change model and assumes that people are taking responsibility for changing their own behaviors, while recognizing ambivalence as part of the process (Table 6.2).

Nonpharmacological methods to increase adherence in psychiatric illnesses

Schizophrenia and psychotic illnesses

As expected, due to its major societal impact and burden (Chapter 1), schizophrenia holds the lion's share of the research on nonpharmacological methods to improve treatment adherence compared to the nonpsychotic illnesses (Table 6.3). Another factor influencing research on nonadherence in schizophrenia is related to the potential effect of insight impairment on treatment adherence (Chapter 3). A review of integrated treatment in schizophrenia shows that medication and psychosocial methods act synergistically: medication is essential in relapse prevention and facilitates involvement in psychosocial treatment, which in turn decreases relapse beyond the effect experienced from medication alone.[15] Of 21 studies comprising 23 nonpharmacological interventions designed to increase antipsychotic medication adherence,[16] the greatest improvement occurred with combinations of educational (knowledge-based), behavioral, and affective (family and individual counseling, supportive home visits) strategies, applied for a median of eight sessions; educational strategies alone were less effective.

Motivational interviewing and the use of the readiness-to-change model can aid in the treatment of dually diagnosed patients. As substance abuse affects approximately half of patients with schizophrenia and when present reduces the

Table 6.2 Principles of motivational interviewing

Goal: increase treatment participation through:

1. Setting realistic treatment expectations
2. Resolving ambivalence
3. Enhancing self efficacy

Motivate for treatment

1. Normalize and amplify doubts
2. Point to discrepancies (where clients are and where they want to be)
3. Support self efficacy
4. Review past treatment experiences
5. Discover potential barriers
6. Summarize sources of nonadherence
7. Involve supportive significant others
8. Provide relevant feedback
9. Break down long term goals into "doable units"
10. Normalize set-backs (change may be imperfect)

Style

1. Open ended questions
2. Empathic assessment
3. Uncover person's beliefs, preferences, expectancies
4. Reflective listening

Adapted from Screening for Alcohol Problems in Social Work Settings. NIAAA Social Work Education, Module 4, (3/04) http://pubs.niaaa.nih.gov/publications/Social/Module4Screening/Module%204%20Screening.ppt

likelihood of medication adherence, there is a dire need for methods to facilitate adherence to substance abuse recovery programs as well as medication adherence. Dually diagnosed psychiatric inpatients were assessed with the University of Rhode Island Change Assessment scale (URICA) (see Adherence Toolkit) and received either standard treatment with medication and psychosocial methods or standard treatment plus motivational interviewing, based on feedback from their URICA scores. Patients who received motivational interviewing had a significantly higher rate of attendance at their first outpatient appointment compared with standard treatment patients.[17]

CBT has been extensively advocated in the treatment of psychosis. The principle that our perception of the environment influences our feelings and behavior has been extensively translated into successful CBT applications for mood and anxiety disorders. The initial step of cognitive therapy in psychosis is to help form an alliance with the patient. Next, therapy attempts to normalize and explain psychotic experiences based on stress vulnerability, focusing on the emotions that may trigger and maintain psychotic symptoms. Other components include exploration of medication attitudes, work on adherence, and facilitating reality testing and ultimately recognition of signs that herald relapse.[12,18]

Jackson and colleagues[19] developed a variation of CBT, Cognitively Oriented Psychotherapy for Early Psychosis (COPE), with a focus on engagement, creating a collaborative work agenda, and addressing adaptation and further morbidity. As cognitive therapy studies in schizophrenia used medication adherence as outcome, compliance therapy developed. This type of therapy incorporates motiva-

Table 6.3 Cognitive and compliance therapy for schizophrenia

Cognitive behavioral therapy for schizophrenia (Turkington 2004[12])	Compliance Therapy (Kemp 1998[13])
• Form alliance	Phase I
• Normalize explanations of psychotic symptoms	• Review illness history
• Formulate case based on stress vulnerability	• Acknowledge negative treatment experiences
• Address:	• Gently inquire of consequences of illness denial
• **Emotions:** that maintain psychotic sympt oms: anger, depression, anxiety	
• **Delusions:** reality testing	
• Hallucinations: diaries, coping strategies, reasoning	
• **Thought disorder:** clarify themes, address emotionally painful topics, use thought linkage	
• **Negative symptoms:** graded activity for affect and cognition	
• Attitude to medication adherence	
• Relapse prevention	
	Phase II
	• Explore ambivalence
	• Address common misconceptions about medication (addiction, loss of self-identity and control)
	• Discuss natural tendency to stop medication when feeling well
	• Elicit inventory of treatment benefits and drawbacks
	• Focus on benefits if any spontaneously identified by patient
	• Use metaphors and create cognitive dissonance
	• Point the disadvantages of noncompliance on lifestyle
	Phase III
	• Normalize treatment using analogies with physical illness
	• Refer to medication as a tool to remain well and reach personal goals
	• Reframe medication as a personal choice to increase quality of life
	• Discuss consequences of stopping medication
	• Discuss prodromal symptoms to target intervention

Table 6.3 (Contd.)	
Cognitive behavioral therapy for schizophrenia (Turkington 2004[12])	**Compliance Therapy (Kemp 1998[13])**
	Phase III
	• Reflective listening
	• Inductive questioning
	• Exploring ambivalence
	• Normalizing
	• Discrepancy between present behavior and broader goals

tional interviewing and cognitive elements to deal with psychotic symptoms, as described by Kemp.[13] In a landmark study, patients with various diagnoses (predominantly schizophrenia or mood disorders) received compliance therapy (see Table 6.3) while hospitalized and were assessed for up to 18 months in the community, where they received care as usual after their hospitalization and initial intervention. Patients' global assessment of function was significantly better and their chance of survival in the community was 2.2 times higher if they received compliance therapy when compared to the control group. The scores on the DAI[20] (see Adherence Toolkit) showed an advantage for patients who received compliance therapy.[13]

In another study, inpatients with various diagnoses had improved scores on the DAI after receiving compliance therapy sessions, but patients with personality disorders, comorbid substance abuse, or more than six prior admissions did not derive benefit from this treatment method.[21] However, Byerly and colleagues[22] found no improvement in antipsychotic adherence measured electronically after a trial of compliance therapy administered to outpatients with schizophrenia or schizoaffective disorder.

Provider characteristics can influence treatment adherence. As previously mentioned, psychiatrists grossly underestimate patients' nonadherence. Once identified, improving adherence may involve adjusting the provider's treatment delivery methods. The therapeutic alliance with the provider can have a significant impact in any type of therapy. A study on the effect of the therapeutic alliance on functional outcome in people with schizophrenia who participated in a CBT-based vocational rehabilitation program showed that people with better alliance with their therapists had better performance in the domains of work quality and personal presentation.[23]

Family treatment delivered by mental health professionals has been proven to increase adherence and prevent relapse in schizophrenia.[24] This therapeutic intervention involves a stepwise process: first, forming an alliance with the patient and family as early in the illness as possible; second, educating families in a group setting about the illness, communication techniques, and problem solving; and third, if necessary, using individualized interventions for each family.[25]

The family-to-family approach uses family members trained as group moderators and has adherence as its end point through maintaining contact with families, keeping them involved and educated. This latter modality was successfully adopted by NAMI in the United States, where it is offered as a 12-week course in multiple locations. NAMI's family-to-family education program was evaluated in a study of 95 families who had been on a waiting list for more than 3 months to enter the program and were assessed for objective and subjective illness burden, depression, and empowerment. The families who received family-to-family program experienced decreased subjective worry and burden of the relative's mental illness and had an increased sense of empowerment regarding the health care system, family, and community, and these gains were maintained 6 months after treatment was completed.[26]

Assertive community treatment (ACT) is a highly intensive treatment program that takes responsibility for the delivery of a broad range of services to mentally ill persons through a team available 24 hours 7 days per week, with the ultimate goals of decreasing hospitalization and increasing quality of life. A review of studies designed to enhance adherence in schizophrenia showed that ACT is a promising adherence tool, although some studies did not describe their methods to assess adherence.[27] When ACT enhanced with family treatment and social skills training was provided to patients with first-episode psychosis, their treatment adherence was significantly higher and psychotic symptoms were significantly lower after 2 years of treatment when compared to patients who received only standard treatment in a mental health center.[28] To add to the controversy as to whether the effects of ACT on the outcome in schizophrenia are mediated through medication adherence versus being an independent effect of the integrated treatment, a Norwegian study showed no effect of integrated treatment on medication adherence in schizophrenia at 2-year follow-up of patients with recent-onset schizophrenia.[29]

Major depression

Although reviews favor cognitive-type approaches to increase adherence in depression treatment, psychoeducation has a role in the treatment of depression, especially in the primary care setting. Educational-type counseling eliciting information about lifestyle and attitudes to treatment and explaining depression and the importance of taking medication increased adherence to antidepressant treatment when applied for only two visits in a group of patients started on tricyclic antidepressants, while treatment leaflets had no effect on patients' adherence with medication.[30] In a long-term study of patients with recurrent major depression, patients assigned to a comprehensive relapse prevention program were offered educational material and two face-to-face and three phone visits with a depression specialist over the first 8 months of treatment and received personalized mail, including the graph of their own self-rated depression scores throughout treatment and checklists of depression symptoms to return to the treatment team. Feedback from the checklists and data on automated medication refills were used to alert the treating primary care doctor when the patient had increased symptomatology or missed refills. Treatment adherence was significantly higher in the intervention group compared to patients who received usual care from their primary care doctors.[31]

Another year-long study in primary care that monitored adherence with MEMS caps showed that patients who were educated on duration of treatment and adverse effects and given information on what to do if problems occurred in treatment had better treatment adherence.[32] In a review of integrated treatment for depression that combined medication with three or four other interventions (care management, educational programs, community-based nurses or pharmacists, telephone contacts), 23 of 28 studies evaluated medication adherence. Of those 23 studies, 15 interventions increased the use of antidepressants by a median of 17.8%.[33]

Bipolar disorder

Cognitive–behavioral therapy, family interventions, interpersonal therapy, and psychoeducation are commonly used in addition to medication in the treatment of bipolar disorder. Frank and colleagues[34] reported on the use of Interpersonal and Social Rhythm Therapy (IPSRT) for acute and maintenance treatment of bipolar patients, compared to acute and maintenance intensive clinical management (ICM) added to medication management, over a 2-year period. IPSRT was developed from interpersonal therapy and its premise implies that unstable daily routines lead to circadian rhythm instability, which can trigger mood episodes in vulnerable people. In turn, stable social routines and interpersonal relationships protect against mood decompensations (Table 6.4).

ICM included education about bipolar illness, medication, its side effects and their management, and sleep hygiene. While adherence with treatment over a 2-year period was not specifically addressed, the study group assigned to IPSRT in the acute and maintenance depressed phase had the lowest attrition, while the groups randomized to ICM in both phases had the highest dropout rate. Patients who received IPSRT added to pharmacological management had longer time before developing a new affective episode. STEP-BD is one of the large-scale multisite studies funded by the NIMH in the United States in an attempt to improve practice guidelines for major mental illnesses. Miklowitz and colleagues[35] reported on a year-long study where patients treated pharmacologically in the acute depression pathway of STEP-BD were randomized to collaborative care, a "control intervention" with three individual sessions focused on reviewing psychoeducational material included in a videotape and workbook given to patients at the onset of the study, CBT, IPSRT, and family-focused therapy. Rates of attrition with each of these modalities are shown in Figure 6.1.

The patients who received intensive psychotherapy had higher rates of clinical recovery at the end of the year than the patients who received collaborative care, and all three types of intensive psychotherapy had comparable outcomes.

A multisite 3-year-long study of more than 300 U.S. VA patients involved psychoeducation, practice according with VA guidelines, and the presence of nurse care coordinators for access, continuity of care, and information flow to

Table 6.4 Interpersonal Social Rhythm Therapy for bipolar disorder[34]

Principles

- Mood symptoms and quality of social relationships and social roles are related
- Maintain daily rhythm, recognize and manage the triggers that disrupt the routines

50 minute sessions

- Identify links between mood symptoms and quality of social roles nad relationships
- Maintain a daily routine
- Resolution of interpersonal problems:
  - Role transitions
  - Interpersonal deficits
  - Grief
  - Disputes
- Manage grief over the potential of a life without bipolar illness

psychiatrist. The duration of manic episodes was reduced by weeks and functioning and quality of life improved as a result of the intervention. The intervention did not differ from usual care in patient retention, as the overall protocol completion rate at 3 years was 80% in both arms of the study.[36]

Integrating substance abuse recovery with medical management

As illustrated in the section on schizophrenia, the interdependence of substance abuse and severe mental illness is prevalent. Project Match,[14] a large U.S. multisite study, compared three types of psychotherapy offered to over 1,500 alcohol-dependent subjects in outpatient or day treatment setting to see if there is any benefit in matching patient attributes with certain types of psychotherapy to enhance the outcome of treatment for alcohol-related disorders. Cognitive–behavioral coping skills therapy was compared with 12-step facilitation therapy and motivational enhancement therapy. At 1-year follow-up, the only subject attribute that differentiated the effectiveness of the three methods of treatment was the severity of the patient's concomitant psychiatric illness. Twelve-step facilitation therapy was more effective for subjects with lower psychiatric severity treatment receiving treatment in an outpatient setting than CBT, whereas no method was superior for patients with high psychiatric severity.

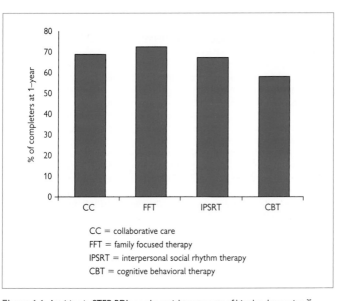

CC = collaborative care
FFT = family focused therapy
IPSRT = interpersonal social rhythm therapy
CBT = cognitive behavioral therapy

Figure 6.1 Attrition in STEP-BD's psychosocial treatments of bipolar depression.[35] (Reprinted from Miklowitz DJ, Otto MW, Frank E, et al. Psychosocial treatments for bipolar depression. A 1-year randomized trial from the Systematic Treatment Enhancement Program. *Archives of General Psychiatry* 2007;64:419–26, with permission from the American Medical Association.)

Various psychosocial treatment methods combined with pharmacological interventions designed to improve abstinence or facilitate engagement in treatment for alcohol and substance use disorders are described in Table 6.5. The outcomes measured in studies comparing psychosocial interventions in substance abuse are heterogeneous in nature, ranging from severity of dependence to treatment dropout, self-reported reduction in alcohol and substance use, and self-reported abstinence.

Ultimately, the minority of patients who seek treatment for alcohol or substance abuse (Chapter 2) benefit equally from existing psychosocial interventions for drug and alcohol cessation, including AA-type self-help programs.[37] In a multisite study of over 2,500 patients with substance abuse disorders at VA hospitals, the dropout rate from 12-step self-help programs at 1-year follow-up after inpatient detoxification was 40%. African American ethnicity, motivation to change, religious background and attendance at religious services, prior 12-step group participation, and social support were protective against dropout. Treatment factors that significantly reduced 12-step self-help dropout rates were already having a sponsor at treatment entry, reading 12-step literature at treatment intake, and being treated in a cohesive, supportive, and spiritually oriented environment.[38]

System-wide barriers and teaching treatment adherence

Practitioners facing constraints of time and service allocation, personnel cuts, and ever-decreasing funding for individual patient visits might quickly consider our remarks in this chapter as out of touch with today's economic reality of psychiatric practice. For example, due to cost, pharmacogenetic tests and high-end techniques to monitor nonadherence (MEMS caps or even a Blackberry communication device) may be impractical; geographical and economic access to a center that combines conventional and alternative medicine may not be feasible for patients and providers. However, health care changes rapidly, and it is certainly possible that our future practice might pay greater attention to medication adherence as a major determinant of treatment outcome.

Should we teach about adherence to trainees in mental health care professions? Per the Liaison Committee on Medical Schools[44] standards, the "faculty and students must demonstrate an understanding of the manner in which people of diverse cultures and belief systems perceive health and illness and respond to various symptoms, diseases, and treatments." Similarly, the American Board of Psychiatry and Neurology mentions in its core competencies that psychiatrists should demonstrate knowledge of "appropriate prescribing practices including age, gender, and ethnocultural variations"[45] and emphasizes the interpersonal and communications skills of the physician, although adherence is not specifically mentioned in any of these documents. Weiden and Rao[3] make a strong case for introducing training on adherence in core residency training in psychiatry and suggest including the following elements, either as a block or as part of psychopharmacology or psychotherapy and psychiatric interviewing courses: definition of adherence, relation with efficacy, assessment, therapeutic alliance, and interventions to improve adherence.

Table 6.5 Psychosocial interventions used in substance abuse research

Intervention	Literature	Outcome
Motivational Enhancement Therapy (MET) Extensive assessment + four treatment sessions over 12 weeks: 1 Personalized feedback about drinking, comparison with a reference group 2 Strenghten committment to change with motivational interviewing techniques based on individual pattient's stage of change 3–4 Review progress, renew motivation and commitment by exploring ambivalence	Project Match Research Group 1997[14] N=952 adults patients with alcohol abuse or dependence in outpatient care N=774 patients in aftercare from inpatient or day treatment	1-year outcome At one year patients attended 1/3 of the sessions of MET, CBT or Twelve-Step facilitation (TSF) offered. All therapies led to significant improvement in drinking outcomes
Twelve Step Facilitation (TSF) is synergistic with Alcoholics Anonymous 12 treatment sessions offered Goals:	Project Match Research Group 1998[39] and Humphreys 1999[40]	3 year outcome 30% of patients were abstinent in Project Match 3years outcome. Patients whose social networks supported drinking had more benefit from TSF than MET. TSF had a slight advantage in drinking outcome at 3 years
Acceptance of: • Alcoholism as a chronic, progressive disease • The fact that patients have lost control of their drinking • The fact that there is no effective cure for alcoholism; only alteranative is abstinence	N>1,700 adult patients with alcohol dependence or abuse	
Surrender: • To a higher power • To follow the AA path for best success		
Interpersonal Cognitive Therapy + pharmacological intervention (buprenorphine in four different dosages) 8 psychotherapy visits offered	Montoya 2005[41] N=90 dually cocaine and heroin dependent adults	Subjects attended 71% of therapy sessions Therapy attendance decreased subsequent drug use most significantly in patients on 16 mg buprenorphine taken every other day

Table 6.5 (Contd.)

Intervention	Literature	Outcome
Phases • Review personal history • Strategies to control drug use • Strengthen skills to prevent use and use resources for support • Separation and termination		
Community Reinforcement approach (CRA) (10 sessions) + naltrexone maintenance (13 psychoprmacological sessions) after detoxification promoted positive reinforcement form individual's real life community context to stimulate medication adherence. Therapy addressed: relationships, drug-refusing behavior, recreational, vocational counseling, problem solving, coping skills and craving management	De Jong 2007[42] N=272 Opioid dependent adults	Patients received 2.5 months of naltrexone Attended 4.3 sessions of psychosocial and 6.6 sessions with psychiatrist 32% abstinence at 16 months
Community reinforcement and family training (CRAFT) = aids family members in modifying the behavior of initially unmotivated adolescent drug and alcohol abusers 12 sessions over 6 months window	Waldron 2007[43] N = 42 parents N = 30 successfully engaged adoles-cents with cannabis abuse	71% of parents were successful in engaging their adolescents in treatment CRAFT improved parent emotional function regardless of engagement of their adolescents in treatment
Phases: • Awareness of negative consequences of drug abuse • Train to reinforce abstinence and reduced substance use • Communication training • Plan activities which interfere with drug use • Increase parents' own drug abstinence reinforcing activities • Prevent dangerousness • Prepare to initiate treatment when adolescent becomes engaged		

References

1. Jayaraman S, Rieder MJ, Matsui DM. Compliance assessment in drug trials: has there been improvement in two decades? *Can J Clin Pharmacol.* 2005;12:e251–253.

2. Langewitz W, Denz M, Keller A, et al. Spontaneous talking time at start of consultation in outpatient clinic: cohort study. *BMJ.* 2002;325:682–683.

3. Weiden PJ, Rao N. Teaching medication compliance to psychiatric residents: placing an orphan topic into a training curriculum. Acad Psychiatry. 2005; 29:203–210.

4. Powell AD. The medication life. *J Psychother Pract Res.* 2001;10:217–222.

5. Deegan PE. The importance of personal medicine: a qualitative study of resilience in people with psychiatric disabilities. *Scand J Public Health Suppl.* 2005;66:29–35.

6. Benedetti F, Mayberg HS, Wager TD, Stohler CS, Zubieta JK. Neurobiological mechanisms of the placebo effect. *J Neurosci.* 2005;25:10390–10402.

7. Goff DC, Cather C, Evins AE, et al. Medical morbidity and mortality in schizophrenia: guidelines for psychiatrists. *J Clin Psychiatry.* 2005;66:183–194.

8. Velligan DI, Gonzales JM. Rehabilitation and recovery in schizophrenia. *Psychiatr Clin North Am.* 2007;30:535–548.

9. Applebaum PS. Assessing Kendra's Law: Five years of outpatient commitment in New York. *Psychiatr Serv.* 2005;56:791–793.

10. Kisely S, Xiao J, Preston N. Impact of compulsory community treatment, on admission rates. Survival analysis using linked mental health and offender databases. *Br J Psychiatry.* 2004;184:432–438.

11. Corrigan PW. Impact of consumer-operated services on empowerment and recovery of people with psychiatric disabilities. *Psychiatr Serv.* 2006;57:1493–1496.

12. Turkington D, Dudley R, Warman D, Beck AT. Cognitive-behavioral therapy for schizophrenia: a review. *J Psychiatr Pract.* 2004;10:5–16.

13. Kemp R, Kirov G, Everitt B, Hayward P, David A. Randomized controlled trial of compliance therapy. 18-month follow-up. *Br J Psychiatry.* 1998;172:413–419.

14. Project MATCH Research Group. Matching alcoholism treatments to client heterogeneity: Project MATCH posttreatment drinking outcomes. *J Stud Alcohol.* 1997;58:7–29.

15. Lenroot R, Bustillo JR, Lauriello J, Keith SJ. Integrated treatment of schizophrenia. *Psychiatr Serv.* 2003;54:1499–1507.

16. Dolder CR, Lacro JP, Leckband S, Jeste DV. Interventions to improve antipsychotic medication adherence: review of recent literature. *J Clin Psychopharmacol.* 2003;23:389–399.

17. Swanson AJ, Pantalon MV, Cohen KR. Motivational interviewing and treatment adherence among psychiatric and dually diagnosed patients. *J Nerv Ment Dis.* 1999;187:630–635.

18. Siddle R, Kingdon D. The management of schizophrenia: cognitive behavioural therapy. *Br J Community Nurs.* 2000;5:20–25.

19. Jackson H, McGorry P, Henry L, et al. Cognitively oriented psychotherapy for early psychosis (COPE): A 1-year follow-up. *Br J Clin Psychol.* 2001;40:57–70.

20. Hogan TP, Awad AG, Eastwood R. A self report scale predictive of drug compliance in schizophrenics: reliability and discriminative validity. *Psychol Med.* 1983;13:177–183.

21. Tay SC. Compliance therapy. An intervention to improve inpatients' attitudes toward treatment. *J Psychosoc Nurs Ment Health Serv*. 2007;45:29–37.

22. Byerly MJ, Fisher R, Carmody T, Rush AJ. A trial of compliance therapy in outpatients with schizophrenia or schizoaffective disorder. *J Clin Psychiatry*. 2005;66:997–1001.

23. Davis LW, Lysaker PH. Therapeutic alliance and improvements in work performance over time in patients with schizophrenia. *J Nerv Ment Dis*. 2007;195:353–357.

24. Leucht S, Heres S. Epidemiology, clinical consequences and psychosocial treatment of nonadherence in schizophrenia. *J Clin Psychiatry*. 2006;67(suppl 5):3–8.

25. McGorry P. Royal Australian and New Zealand College of Psychiatrists Clinical practice guidelines for the treatment of schizophrenia and related disorders. *Aust N Z J Psychiatry*. 2005;39:1–30.

26. Dixon L, Lucksted A, Stewart B, et al. Outcomes of the peer-taught 12-week family-to-family education program for severe mental illness. *Acta Psychiatr Scand*. 2004;109:207–215.

27. Zygmunt A, Olfson M, Boyer CA, Mechanic D. Interventions to improve medication adherence in schizophrenia. *Am J Psychiatry*. 2002;159:1653–1664.

28. Petersen L, Jeppesen P, Thorup A, et al. A randomised multicentre trial of integrated versus standard treatment for patients with a first episode of psychotic illness. *BMJ*. 2005;331:602.

29. Morken G, Grawe RW, Widen JH. Effects of integrated treatment on antipsychotic medication adherence in a randomized trial in recent-onset schizophrenia. *J Clin Psychiatry*. 2007;68:566–571.

30. Peveler R, George C, Kinmonth AL, Campbell M, Thomson C. Effect of antidepressant drug counselling and information leaflets on adherence to drug treatment in primary care: randomised controlled trial. *BMJ*. 1999;319:612–615.

31. Katon W, Rutter C, Ludman EJ, et al. A randomized trial of relapse prevention of depression in primary care. *Arch Gen Psychiatry*. 2001;58:241–247.

32. Brown C, Battista DR, Sereika S, Bruehlman RD, Dunbar-Jacob J, Thase ME. How can you improve antidepressant adherence? *J Fam Pract*. 2007; 56:356–363.

33. Williams JW, Gerrity M, Holsinger T, Dobscha S, Gaynes B, Dietrich A. Systematic review of multifaceted interventions to improve depression care. *Gen Hosp Psychiatry*. 2007;29:91–116.

34. Frank E, Kupfer DJ, Thase ME, et al. Two-year outcomes for interpersonal and social rhythm therapy in individuals with bipolar I disorder. *Arch Gen Psychiatry*. 2005;62:996–1004.

35. Miklowitz DJ, Otto MW, Frank E, et al. Psychosocial treatments for bipolar depression. A 1-year randomized trial from the Systematic Treatment Enhancement Program. *Arch Gen Psychiatry*. 2007;64:419–426.

36. Bauer MS, McBride L, Williford WO, et al. Collaborative care for bipolar disorder: Part II. Impact on clinical outcome, function and costs. *Psychiatr Serv*. 2006;57:937–945.

37. Ferri M, Amato L, Davoli M. Alcoholics Anonymous and other 12-step programmes for alcohol dependence. *Cochrane Database Syst Rev*. 2006; 3:CD005032.

38. Kelly JF, Moos R. Drop-out form 12-step self-help groups: prevalence, predictors and counteracting treatment influences. *J Subst Abuse Treat*. 2003;24:241–250.

39. Project MATCH Research Group. Matching alcoholism treatments to client heterogeneity: Project MATCH three-year drinking outcomes. *Alcohol Clin Exp Res.* 1998;22:1300–1311.

40. Humphreys K. Professional interventions that facilitate 12-step self-help group involvement. Alcohol Res Health. 1999;23:93–98.

41. Montoya ID, Schroeder JR, Preston KL, et al. Influence of psychotherapy attendance on buprenorphine treatment outcome. *J Subst Abuse Treat.* 2005; 28:247–254.

42. De Jong CA, Roozen HG, van Rossum LGM, et al. High abstinence rates in heroin addicts by a new comprehensive treatment approach. *Am J Addict.* 2007;16:124–130.

43. Waldron HB, Kern-Jones S, Turner C, Peterson TR, Ozechowski TJ. Engaging resistant adolescents in drug abuse treatment. *J Subst Abuse Treat.* 2007;32:133–142.

44. Liaison Committee on Medical Education. *Standards for Accreditation of Medical Education Programs Leading to the M.D. Degree,* June 2008. http://www.lcme.org/functions2008jun.pdf. Accessed July 25, 2008.

45. American Board of Psychiatry & Neurology, Psychiatry and Neurology Core Competencies, Version 4.1. http://www.abpn.com/downloads/core_comp_outlines/core_psych_neuro_v4.1.pdf

Appendix

Appendix

Psychiatric adherence toolkit

The psychiatric adherence toolkit includes:

- Useful Web sites
- Labs performing AmpliChip analysis of polymorphisms in CYP450 2D6 and 2C19
- Medication monitoring systems
- Adherence rating scales

Useful Web sites

National Alliance on Mental Illness (NAMI): www.nami.org
NAMI Family-to-Family program: http://www.nami.org/Template.cfm?
  Section=Family-to-Family&Template=/TaggedPage/TaggedPageDisplay.
  cfm&TPLID=4&ContentID=39771
Depression and Bipolar Support Alliance (DBSA): http://www.dbsalliance.org
Mental Health America: www.mentalhealthamerica.net
LCME standards: http://www.lcme.org/functions2008jun.pdf

Labs performing AmpliChip analysis of polymorphisms in CYP450 2D6 and 2C19

Laboratory	Contact information
Affymetrix Clinical Services Lab	diagnosticsales@affymetrix.com
Center for Molecular Medicine	www.cmmdx.org/physicians, 616-391-4325
Georgia Esoteric and Molecular Lab, LLC	www.gamolecularlab.com, 706-721-5116
LabCorp	www.labcorp.com, 800-533-0567
Specialty Laboratories	www.specialtylabs.com, 800-421-4449
Spectrum Laboratories	spectrumlab.com, 888-664-7601
UCI Pathology Services	888-UCI-LABS

Medication monitoring systems

Information Mediary Corporation
Med-ic® Electronic Compliance Moniter© (http://med-ic.biz/medicecm.shtml)
eCAP™ (http://ecap.biz)
Tel: 613–745-8400
inquiry@informationmediary.com

AARDEX Group
The MEMS® cap
www.aardexgroup.com
Tel: 877–227-3391
Info-usa@aardexgroup.com

INRange Systems, Inc
EMMA™ System
www.inrangesystems.com
Tel: 814–940-1870

Interactive Medical Developments, LC
MD.2™
www.imd2.com
Tel: 877–563-2632
haroldp@imp2.com

PsytronRx
Varied monitoring equipment
www.psytronrx.com
Tel: 734–347-1462

Adherence rating scales

Adherence rating scales can be very useful tools in the context of clinical care. While there are a number of adherence rating scales available, the choice of adherence rating scale should be based on feasibility and usefulness in the specific clinical setting.

APPENDIX A

SAMPLE ITEMS FROM BRIEF MEDICATION QUESTIONNAIRE (**)

1. Please list below all of the medications you took in the PAST WEEK. For each medication you list, please answer each of the questions in the box below.

IN THE PAST WEEK:						
a. Medication name and strength	b. How many days did you take it?	c. How many times per day did you take it?	d. How many pills did you take each time?	e. How many times did you miss taking a pill?	f. For what reason were you taking it?	g. How well does the medicine work for you? 1 = well 2 = okay 3 = not well

_____ ___ ___ ___ ___ _____ ___
_____ ___ ___ ___ ___ _____ ___
_____ ___ ___ ___ ___ _____ ___

APPENDIX A (CONT.)

2. Do any of your medications bother you in any way? YES _____ NO _____

   a. IF YES, please name the medication and check below how much it bothers you.

How much did it bother you?

Medication name	A lot	Some	A little	Never	In what way did it bother you?
_____	___	___	___	___	_____
_____	___	___	___	___	_____
_____	___	___	___	___	_____

3. Below is a list of problems that people sometimes have with their medicines. Please check how hard it is for you to do each of the following:

	Very hard	Somewhat hard	Not hard at all	COMMENT (Which medicine)
a. Open or close the medication bottle	___	___	___	_____
b. Read the print on the bottle	___	___	___	_____
c. Remember to take all the pills	___	___	___	_____
d. Get your refills in time	___	___	___	_____
e. Take so many pills at the same time	___	___	___	_____

(**) The original copyrighted instrument is available from the first author.

SCORING PROCEDURES FOR BMQ SCREENS

Screen	Scoring	
Regimen Screen (Questions 1a–1e)		
Did R fail to list the prescribed drug in the initial (spontaneous) report?	1 = yes	0 = no
Did R stop or interrupt therapy due to a late refill or other reason?	1 = yes	0 = no
Did R report any missed days or doses?	1 = yes	0 = no
Did R reduce or cut down the prescribed amount per dose?	1 = yes	0 = no
Did R take any extra doses or more medication than prescribed?	1 = yes	0 = no
Did R report "don't know" in response to any questions?	1 = yes	0 = no
Did R refuse to answer any questions?	1 = yes	0 = no
NOTE: Score of ≥1 indicates positive screen for potential nonadherence.		
Belief Screen (Questions 1g and 2–2a)		
Did R report "not well" or "don't know" in response to Q 1g?	1 = yes	0 = no
Did R name the prescribed drug as a drug that bothers him/her?	1 = yes	0 = no
NOTE: Score of ≥1 indicates positive screen for belief barriers		
Recall Screen (Questions 1c and 3c)		
Did R receive a multiple dose regimen (2 or more times/day)?	1 = yes	0 = no
Did R report "very hard" or "somewhat hard" in response to Q 3c?	1 = yes	0 = no
NOTE: Score of ≥1 indicates positive screen for recall barriers		

R = respondent

*Copyright: Corresponding author. Tel.: +1 608 2652128; fax: +1 608 2623397; e-mail: blsvarstad@pharmacy.wisc.edu)
Svarstad BL et al. The Brief Medication Questionnaire: a tool for screening patient adherence and barriers to adherence. Patient Educ Couns 1999;37:113-24.

Figure AP.1 Brief Medication Questionnaire (BMQ). (Reprinted from Svarstad BL, et al. The Brief Medication Questionnaire: a tool for screening patient adherence and barriers to adherence. *Patient Education Counseling* 1999;37:113–24, with permission from Elsevier.)

BRIEF ADHERENCE RATING SCALE

Information obtained from patient:

1. How many pills of _____ (name of antipsychotic) did the doctor tell you to take each day?	
2. Over the month since your last visit with me, on how many days did you NOT TAKE your _____ (name of antipsychotic)?	Few, if any (<7)
	7–13
	14–20
	Most (>20)
3. Over the month since your last visit with me, on how many days did you TAKE LESS THAN the prescribed number of pills of your _____ (name of antipsychotic)?	Always/Almost always (76–100% of the time) = 1
	Usually (51–75% of the time) = 2
Note: 1 = poor adherence 4 = good adherence	Sometimes (26–50% of the time) = 3
	Never/Almost never (0–25% of the time) = 4

Please place a single verticle line on the dotted line that you believe best describes, out of the prescribed antipsychotic medication (_____) doses, the proportion of doses taken by the patient in the past month.

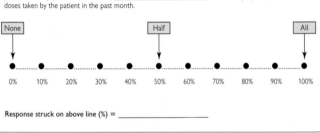

Response struck on above line (%) = _____

Figure AP.2 Brief Adherence Rating Scale (BARS). (Reprinted from Byerly MJ et al. The Brief Adherence Rating Scale (BARS) validated against electronic monitoring in assessing the antipsychotic medication adherence of outpatients with schizophrenia and schizoaffective disorder. Schizophrenia Resource 2008;100:60–9, with permission from Elsevier.)

Table AP.1 Medication Adherence Questionnaire (MAQ)

	Corrected Item-to-total Correlation
1. Do you ever forget to take your medicine?	0.515
2. Are you careless at times about taking your medicine?	0.479
3. When you feel better do you sometimesstop taking your medicine?	0.527
4. Sometimes if you feel worse when you take the medicine, do you stop taking it?	0.561
Scoring: high–low; Yes = 0; No = 1	
Range: 0–4	
Mean weighted: n = 290; $\bar{X}$ = 2.31	
Cronbach alpha: 0.61	

Reprinted with permission from Morisky DE et al. Concurrent and predictive validity of a self-reported measure of medication adherence. *Med Care* 1986;24:67–74, with permission from Lippincott, Williams & Wilkins.

Table AP.2 The Medication Adherence Rating Scale (MARS)

Please respond to the following statements by circling the answer which best describes your behaviour or the attitude you have held toward your medication in the past week.

1. Do you ever forget to take your medication? Yes/No
2. Are you careless at times about taking your medicine? Yes/No
3. When you feel better, do you sometimes stop taking your medicine? Yes/No
4. Sometimes if you feel worse when you take the medicine, do you stop taking it? Yes/No
5. I take my medication only when I am sick. Yes/No
6. It is unnatural for my mind and body to be controlled by medication. Yes/No
7. My thoughts are clearer on medication. Yes/No
8. By staying on medication, I can prevent getting sick. Yes/No
9. I feel weird, like a 'zombie', on medication. Yes/No
10. Medication makes me feel tired and sluggish. Yes/No

Reprinted with permission from Thompson K, et al. Reliability and validity of a new Medication Adherence Rating Scale (MARS) for the psychoses. *Schizophr Res.* 2000;42:241–247, with permission from Elsevier.

Table AP.3: Drug Attitude Inventory (DAI-30)

1. I don't need to take medication once I feel better	T F
2. For me, the good things about medication outweigh the bad	T F
3. I feel strange, "doped up", on medication	T F
4. Even when I am not in hospital I need medication regularly	T F
5. If I take medication, it's only because of pressure from other people	T F
6. I am more aware of what I am doing, of what is going on around me, when I am on medication	T F
7. Taking medications will do me no harm	T F
8. I take medications of my own free choice	T F
9. Medications make me feel more relaxed	T F
10. I am no different on or off medication	T F
11. The unpleasant effects of medication are always present	T F
12. Medication makes me feel tired and sluggish	T F
13. I take medication only when I feel ill	T F
14. Medications are slow-acting poisons	T F
15. I get along better with people when I am on medication	T F
16. I can't concentrate on anything when I am taking medication	T F
17. I know better than the doctors when to stop taking medication	T F
18. I feel more normal on medication	T F
19. I would rather be ill then taking medication	T F
20. It is unnatural for my mind and body to be controlled by medications	T F
21. My thoughts are clearer on medication	T F
22. I should keep taking medication even if I feel well	T F
23. Taking medication will prevent me from having a breakdown	T F
24. It is up to the doctor to decide when I should stop taking medication	T F
25. Things that I could do easily are much more difficult when I am on medication	T F
26. I am happier and feel better when I am taking medications	T F
27. I am given medication to control behaviour that other people (not myself) don't like	T F
28. I can't relax on medication	T F
29. I am in better control of myself when taking medication	T F
30. By staying on medications I can prevent myself getting sick	T F

Adapted from "A self-report scale predictive of drug compliance in schizophrenics: reliability and discriminative validity", Hogan TP, Awad AG, Eastwood R, *Psychological Medicine* 1983, 13, 177–183, with permission from Cambridge University Press.

Table AP.4 Rating of Medication Influences (ROMI)

Part I: Reasons for Adherence

"Are you (considering) taking your medication because.....	DEGREE OF INFLUENCE		
AD 1. **PERCEIVED DAILY BENEFIT**	1	2	3
You believe the medicine helps you feel better?	None	Mild	Strong
AD 2. **FEAR OF RELAPSE**	1	2	3
You believe taking medication prevents your illness or symptoms from returning?	None	Mild	Strong
AD 3. **SIDE EFFECT RELIEF**	1	2	3
Compared with other medicines, this one has fewer side effects so it is easier for to stay on it?	None	Mild	Strong
AD 4. **FULFILLMENT OF LIFE GOALS**	1	2	3
What are your goals? Do you feel that medication helps you achieve your goals?	None	Mild	Strong
AD 5. **DEFERENCE TO AUTHORITY**	1	2	3
You do what the doctor tells you?	None	Mild	Strong
AD 6. **POSITIVE RELATION WITH CLINICAL STAFF**	1	2	3
You are influenced by someone whose opinion is important to you?	None	Mild	Strong
AD 7. **OUTSIDE POSITIVE OPINION ABOUT TAKING MEDICATIONS**	1	2	3
Does someone in your family or a friend believe that you should be taking medicine?	None	Mild	Strong
AD 8. **OUTSIDE OPINION THAT CURRENT MEDICATION IS BETTER**	1	2	3
Does someone you know tell you that the medicine you are taking now is better than previous medications?	None	Mild	Strong
AD 9. **OUTSIDE PRESSURE/FORCE**	1	2	3
Are you being pressured or forced to take medication by someone?	None	Mild	Strong

Part II: Reasons for Nonadherence

"Are you reluctant to take your medication because......."	DEGREE OF INFLUENCE		
NAD10. **NO DAILY BENEFIT**	1	2 Mild	3
You don't feel any better after taking the medication?	None		Strong
NAD11. **MEDICATIONS CURRENTLY UNNECESSARY**	1	2	3
Although you may have needed them in the past, you don't currently need the medication?	None	Mild	Strong
NAD12. **NEVER WAS ILL**	1	2	3
You don't believe you ever had a mental illness (emotional problem) that needs medications?	None	Mild	Strong
NAD13. **INTERFERES WITH LIFE GOALS**	1	2	3
You feel that medication interferes with achieving certain goals or life aspirations?	None	Mild	Strong

Table AP.4 (Contd.)

NAD14. DISTRESSED BY SIDE EFFECTS	1	2	3
The side effects of the medicine are too upsetting to you?	None	Mild	Strong
NAD15. EMBARRASSMENT OR STIGMA OVER MEDS/ILLNESS	1	2	3
You feel embarrassed about taking medication?	None	Mild	Strong
NAD16. CHANGE IN APPEARANCE	1	2	3
You look "medicated" to other people?	None	Mild	Strong
NAD17. OUTSIDE OPPOSITION TO TAKING MEDICATIONS	1	2	3
Someone in your family or a friend believes that you should not be taking medicine?	None	Mild	Strong
NAD18. TREATMENT ACCESS PROBLEMS	1	2	3
You have difficulty getting to your appointments, and/or difficulty getting meds?	None	Mild	Strong
NAD19. SUBSTANCE ABUSE	1	2	3
Do you stop your medications before you drink or get high, or during times that you use?	None	Mild	Strong

Reprinted with permission from Weiden P, et al. Rating of medication influences (ROMI) scale in schizophrenia. *Schizophr Bull.* 1994;20:297–310.

Table AP.5 Stages of Change Questionnaire (URICA-University of Rhode Island Change Assessment)

Precontemplation

Item:

1. As far as I'm concerned, I don't have any problems that need changing.

5. I'm not the problem one. It doesn't make sense for me to be here.

11. Being here is pretty much of a waste of time for me because the problem doesn't have to do with me.

13. I guess I have faults, but there's nothing that I really need to change.

23. I may be part of the problem, but I don't really think I am.

26. All this talk about psychology is boring. Why can't people just forget about their problems?

29. I have worries but so does the next person. Why spend time thinking about them?

31. I would rather cope with my faults than try to change them.

Contemplation

Item:

2. I think I might be ready for some self-improvement.

4. It might be worthwhile to work on my problem.

8. I've been thinking that I might want to change something about myself.

12. I'm hoping this place will help me to better understand myself.

15. I have a problem and I really think I should work on it.

19. I wish I had more ideas on how to solve my problem.

21. Maybe this place will be able to help me.

24. I hope that someone here will have some good advice for me.

Table AP.5 (Contd.)

Action

Item:

3. I am doing something about the problems that had been bothering me.

7. I am finally doing some work on my problems.

10. At times my problem is difficult, but I'm working on it.

14. I am really working hard to change.

17. Even though I'm not always successful in changing, I am at least working on my problem.

20. I have started working on my problems but I would like help.

25. Anyone can talk about changing; I'm actually doing something about it.

30. I am actively working on my problem.

Maintenance

Item:

6. It worries me that I might slip back on a problem I have already changed, so I am here to seek help.

9. I have been successful in working on my problem but I'm not sure I can keep up the effort on my own.

16. I'm not following through with what I had already changed as well as I had hoped, and I'm here to prevent a relapse of the problem.

18. I thought once I had resolved the problem I would be free of it, but sometimes I still find myself struggling with it.

22. I may need a boost right now to help me maintain the changes I've already made.

27. I'm here to prevent myself from having a relapse of my problem.

28. It is frustrating, but I feel I might be having a recurrence of a problem I thought I had resolved.

32. After all I had done to try to change my problem, every now and again it comes back to haunt me.

Reprinted from McConnaughy EN, et al. Stages of change in psychotherapy: measurement and sample profiles. *Psychotherapy: Theory, Research and Practice.* 1983;20:368–375, with permission from University of Rhode Island, Cancer Research and Prevention Center.

Index

Page numbers ending with an *f* indicate a figure; with a *t* a table.

103

Notes

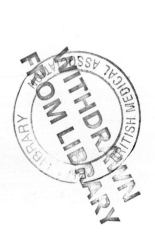